A Map of the Child

A Map
of the
Child

A PEDIATRICIAN'S
TOUR OF THE BODY

Darshak Sanghavi

A John Macrae Book
HENRY HOLT AND COMPANY   NEW YORK

Owl Books
Henry Holt and Company, LLC
Publishers since 1866
175 Fifth Avenue
New York, New York 10010
www.henryholt.com

An Owl Book® and ® are registered trademarks of
Henry Holt and Company, LLC.

Library of Congress Cataloging-in-Publication Data

Sanghavi, Darshak.
　　A map of the child : a pediatrician's tour of the body / Darshak Sanghavi.—1st ed.
　　　p.　cm.
　　Includes index.
　　ISBN-13: 978-0-8050-7511-3
　　ISBN-10: 0-8050-7511-9
　　1. Sanghavi, Darshak.　2. Pediatricians—United States—Biography.　I. Title.
RJ43.S26 A3 2003
618.92'00092—dc21　　　　　　　　2002027489
[B]

Henry Holt books are available for special promotions and
premiums. For details contact: Director, Special Markets.

First published in hardcover in 2003 by Henry Holt
First Owl Books Edition 2004

DESIGNED BY KELLY S. TOO

Printed in the United States of America

3　5　7　9　10　8　6　4　2

For my father,
Mahendra Sanghavi

The stories in this book are true. To preserve confidentiality, however, the names and certain identifying details of the patients, families, and health care personnel (with the exception of those in the latter part of the chapter about bones) have been changed.

CONTENTS

Preface: A Life Begins

Water diffuses so slowly, I remember thinking, as fluid entered the window of the thin plastic wand. Home pregnancy tests, like the one my wife, Elizabeth, was using, detect a hormone called human chorionic gonadotropin, or HCG. The placenta, which connects a mother's circulation to her developing child's, produces the telltale HCG of which a trace escapes into the urine. Pregnancy tests are exquisitely sensitive; they can detect the hormone at the approximate concentration of a teaspoon dissolved in an Olympic-size swimming pool.

In the window, the reaction began as a blush of red slowly coalesced into a shape. Elizabeth drew a sharp breath as the pregnancy test revealed an answer, and turned to me with misted eyes. The wand had a small positive sign in the window. With her green eyes and ringlets of red hair, Elizabeth has an otherworldly ability to cast spells over me. We're a good match. She's a science teacher, a devotee of flasks and dissections and food webs, but she also believes in ghosts and magic. Now we'd be parents together.

My wife was about four weeks pregnant and our child was the size of a grain of rice. We eagerly opened one of my old medical school textbooks and read about the development of a baby's tiny heart, lungs, and brain. We relished words like *notochord*, *branchial arches*, and *gastrulation*.

At the same time, I began to worry like many parents about our new child. Would he or she arrive with a healthy, well-functioning body? Would our baby develop any serious illnesses during infancy? Would there be problems hidden away that would appear only later, as our child entered nursery school or went off to summer camp?

As a pediatrician, I often field questions from anxious mothers and fathers concerned about the health of their children. After learning I'd be a father, though, I realized that parents of my patients weren't just apprehensive, they were often genuinely curious. I recalled that when my wife's pregnancy test came up positive, my first impulse had been to find a textbook and review how a baby's body forms from an embryo. Perhaps, like myself and many other parents, you share this fascination and want to understand more about the bodies of children.

The following chapters are a crash course in anatomy, physiology, public health policy, the culture of medicine, and child psychology—but at the same time, not a set of lectures. Instead, they're a collection of stories. Pediatric medicine is explored, with a continuing sense of wonder, through narratives of children and families dealing with illness.

How best should one investigate the body of a child? My own medical training, or residency, consisted of rotations spent caring for specific body parts. One month I took care of lungs, the next hearts, then kidneys, and so on. Like a residency, this book takes the form of a medical tour. Each narrative chapter involves a different organ system: the first explores a child's lungs, the next deals with the heart, and so on through chapters about blood, bones, brain, skin, gonads, and the gut.

To understand the lungs' development, for example, we meet a premature infant born before his lungs were fully formed and see the treatment that saved his life. In another chapter, a girl who grows too fast and sees ghosts leads us on to an exploration of the brain's anatomy. Later, we discover how gender develops in the fetus in the case of a girl who wasn't quite a girl at birth. These and other unusual cases are used to explore the inner workings of the developing body. However, common pediatric issues aren't neglected. Along the way, you'll also learn—among many other things—why some infants get diaper rashes, what causes pneumonia, how broken bones heal, what vitamins pregnant women need, and how attention deficit disorder is diagnosed. Controversial areas in child health are also covered, drawing on medical history, recent research, and personal experience in discussions of circumcision, vaccination for chicken pox, child abuse, alternative medicine, birth control for adolescents, and other divisive topics.

In addition to satisfying curiosity, medical knowledge also offers comfort to parents and children confronted by sickness. Just weeks before my wife learned she was pregnant with our baby, I sat a prolonged vigil in an intensive care unit where my father lay critically ill. Looking at my father's unseeing face was bearable since I knew the doctors continuously infused his veins with fentanyl, a narcotic similar to morphine. This small molecule bound his neurons and gave him merciful sleep, undisturbed by the tubes and machines invading his body. I thought about my father often in the time that followed.

Though medical knowledge expanded my happiness when I learned I'd be a father, it also offered me solace when my own father was ill. This book thus was written with the hope that understanding medicine and disease can itself be healing. Coming to terms with illness, especially in one's own family, isn't easy. As we consider technical aspects of medicine in the following pages, we'll also observe the struggles of parents and children in extraordinary circumstances. Though a family's experience with disease can be unpredictable, even erratic, certain themes have appeared repeatedly, I've found in my work as a pediatrician. Each chapter of this book focuses both on an organ and on one of these motifs—for example, the need for forgiveness, the sorrow of loss, or the power of perseverance—to which I allude in the chapter's subtitle.

My own story as a doctor has centered on the care of children. After completing an undergraduate degree at Harvard, I attended medical school at Johns Hopkins, and then returned to Harvard to train at Children's Hospital in Boston. I've practiced medicine in a variety of settings including Japan, Peru, Kenya, India, and Appalachia, and most recently in the Navajo reservation as a pediatrician for the U.S. Indian Health Service. Although I've published scientific papers on topics ranging from the molecular biology of cell death to tuberculosis transmission patterns in Peruvian slums, my attention has always returned to children and their health. I returned to Boston and Children's Hospital, in pediatric cardiology, in September of 2002.

Our exploration will begin with the lungs of a child and one night in Bombay.

~ 1 ~

Lungs

FROM BOMBAY TO BOSTON, STORIES OF
PEOPLE AND LUNGS SEEKING FREEDOM

The summer before beginning medical school I visited India, the land my mother fled almost twenty-two years earlier while pregnant with me, her first child. She found her new husband's extended family so fixed on enforcing decayed social rules ("Always walk with your head bowed. Never address the in-laws directly. No laughing is allowed.") that she felt suffocated, and one day talked my father into a new life in the United States. As I grew up, my family visited Bombay perhaps every four years and noted a gradual clearing in the social atmosphere that hung like smog over my father's homestead.

Still, I preferred the company of my mother's side of the family during our sojourns, and I often spent nights in the Dadar district outside Bombay, where my mother's sister lived with her four adult children. Crammed into the three-bedroom apartment, the youngest family members (myself included) slept on feather cots in the living room. Here my troubles began. Every night for almost three weeks, I descended into an airless world where breathing could no longer be taken for granted.

One night, I arose from the bedding and walked over to the window, skirting three of my cousins who were sleeping soundly on the stone floor. Gazing over the indigo night of Bombay, I was overwhelmed by waves of coughing. I leaned out the window, closed my eyes, and began to hack violently. The sounds echoed from the stucco houses along the street. Every breath was a struggle. Indeed, my chest had a new definition of muscles toned by my nightly labors.

Breathing is fundamentally passive. No part of the body pushes air into the lungs; instead, by reducing the pressure in the chest, one coaxes in air. Breathing is an act of physical negotiation where one entices air from the atmosphere into a low-pressure area. I braced my arms against the ledge and inhaled deeply. Just below my rib cage, a bell-shaped muscle, the diaphragm, flattened, creating a vacuum in my thorax. Like an opening bellows, my lungs began pulling air through the mouth and nose.

Never having considered breathing a complicated activity, I realized how every breath was a series of small steps. Air entered my mouth, passed teeth and the tonsils' arches, and proceeded to the back of the throat. There, the beginnings of breath merged with air from the nose, where moist membranes humidified and warmed the air. The combined air flowed down to the base of the tongue, a half-inch down from the tonsils. The breath then came to a crossroads where it could either proceed down the esophagus or enter an open portal called the trachea. Because the area of low pressure was in the trachea the air went there, past a flap called the epiglottis. At this point the air was at the Adam's apple, or thyroid cartilage, which provides a scaffold for the trachea. The air had entered the lungs.

From the trachea, the air branched into tubular air spaces called bronchi and then smaller bronchioles and then finally to hair-thin byways called alveoli. Tiny blood vessels run parallel to the alveoli, and a membrane only one cell thick separates the two areas. Oxygen percolates from air into the blood, and carbon dioxide returns. As the breath finished, my diaphragm returned elastically to its bell shape, and the spent air was pushed out with a low-pitched, wheezing sound.

Exhausted, I fantasized about the ideal breath, one that allowed pure air to flow effortlessly. But my reverie was interrupted by another spasm of coughing and this time I brought up brown, jelly-like sputum.

I returned to my bedding. (Months later in the United States a physician explained that the bedding contained dust, the instigator of my distress. That's why the symptoms came at night.) Because sleeping on a single pillow was intolerable, I had placed three pillows under my head and concentrated on my respirations. Breathe out, breathe in, breathe out, and breathe in, I said to myself. After a while, the feeling of iron bands around my chest relented somewhat. A temporary calm came, the closest thing to sleep I felt.

Years later, I tried to sleep in a call room at the Brigham and Women's Hospital, when my pager went off. Two weeks earlier, I had begun a rotation in the newborn intensive care unit, or NICU, at "the Brigham," a sister hospital just a block from my home base at Boston Children's Hospital. The pager went off every time there was a high-risk delivery in the obstetrics unit downstairs.

I grabbed the bright yellow tackle box that held everything needed for resuscitation, and sprinted for the fourth time that day through the NICU, past Zelda the secretary who called out "Operating room four" (the location of the delivery), around the corner, and down the stairs one flight. On the way, I mentally replayed the resuscitation techniques in my head, reviewing the proper-size tubes to be placed in premature infants' windpipes if needed, dosages of medications to be given if the heartbeat was slow, and the method of administering chest compressions. The latter was particularly different from the method used on adults; instead of using a full palm, one used only two fingers placed on the newborn's chest, pushing down less than an inch to pump a heart the size of a small plum.

In the operating room vestibule I met Mary, the NICU nurse assigned to the case. Already wearing surgical scrubs, we quickly donned shoe covers, face masks, and bouffant surgical caps, then slipped on latex gloves before entering the operating room. A delivery in the operating room meant we were probably dealing with an emergency cesarean birth, which often meant that the fetus was in distress and needed emergency delivery. "Thanks for coming," said an operating room nurse, not looking up from her clipboard. "Your setup is there," she added, gesturing to the far right of the theater.

The first time I saw a live birth in medical school, I earned an amused smile from the supervising resident when tears rolled down my face. Childbirth never ceased to amaze me, and my eyes would frequently mist, a condition I handled by blinking rapidly. This time I wouldn't have time to hide my tears. Justine Flax, a thirty-two-year-old woman, was about to give birth to twins, the product of test tube fertilization. The trouble was, they were being born about two months too early. Justine had named them already; the first-born would be Adam, and he would be mine to resuscitate if necessary. I couldn't see the mother's face when I entered the suite; a sterile surgical partition divided her neck from her body, obscuring us from each other's view. Introductions would have to wait.

Before getting any further information, I opened up my tackle box to lay out my equipment. Obstetricians are notorious for suddenly delivering a baby when the occasion requires it; the fastest cesarean delivery I ever saw was accomplished in less than sixty seconds from the woman's entrance into the operating room.

The tackle box can tell you a lot about a resident's personality, since its organization carries a characteristic imprint. Methodical residents place their tubes, solutions, and needles in an orderly array. Those that are sure of their skills gradually open and prepare fewer tubes, while less confident ones open several because they anticipate making mistakes. (I would be chilled if a resident laid out five windpipe tubes for my own child's delivery; that would mean he's lousy at placing them correctly.) I took particular pride in organizing my tackle box. From it, I extracted a small 2.5 French tube, the smallest in the box. "French" refers to the size of the tube, but to me the term "French tubes" has always connoted some exotic pastry.

The tube was critical because Adam's tiny lungs weren't ready to breathe at this stage. Like seedlings, Adam's lungs sprouted from his gastrointestinal tract when he was only one month in the womb. At the time, Adam himself was a ball of cells smaller than a pea. All of his internal organs began as microscopic pouches growing out of what eventually became the skin, in a sort of human origami. First came the gastrointestinal system, initially a microscopic tube with no identifiable mouth or stomach or intestines. In turn, a swelling of this tube gave rise to the lungs.

The lungs are a spectacular solution to a fundamental physical problem: How does an organism get enough oxygen from the air to each of its billions of cells? Without lungs, we might all look like sea kelp, a type of algae that never developed a respiratory system, and continues to grow in two dimensions, up to one hundred fifty feet long and several inches wide but only a few hairs thick. Requiring oxygen just as humans do, the sea kelp must position every cell of its body near a source of it. Every cell, solitary in its respiration, communes directly with the atmosphere. In contrast, complex organisms like humans have thickness and volume, necessitating a distribution scheme for oxygen to cells deep in the body. Lungs allow us to become three-dimensional, since they collect oxygen for the blood, which serves as transport to bodily regions far from the light of the sun and the breezes of oxygen. Lest we humans develop an undue hubris, Vance Tucker of Duke University has demonstrated that at an altitude of 18,000 feet, sparrows still fly with no problem, whereas mice and humans quickly require supplemental oxygen. In contrast to mammals, birds have unidirectional airflow through the lungs, allowing superior oxygen extraction from air.

Oxygen turbocharges our highly evolved cells, allowing them to extract ten times more energy than their primitive ancestors, called prokaryotes. Biologist Lynn Margulis has hypothesized that a few billion years ago a prokaryote engulfed another organism called a mitochondrion. The two cells cooperated: the prokaryote housed the mitochondrion, which produced energy for its host at a phenomenal rate by using oxygen. It was the start of a beautiful friendship that continues to this day in our cells.

Complex organisms depend on this so-called aerobic respiration, in which mitochondria combine oxygen with nutrients, literally burning food. Without oxygen, our cells become primitive again like the cells of billions of years ago, capable only of paltry metabolic feats. When muscles burn after vigorous activity, the pain means they were briefly oxygen starved and therefore accumulated lactic acid. Muscles recover quickly, since the acid is neutralized once activity ends. Brain tissue, though, is not so forgiving and can withstand oxygen deprivation only for a few minutes before suffering permanent damage. In essence, the development of aerobic respiration also made suffocation possible. This was the problem Adam Flax was about to face.

Adam's mother, Justine, had premature labor, meaning that her uterus began contractions far too early. The uterus is something like *good analogy*

a heart, except that instead of blood it pumps a baby. The uterus begins contracting slowly, squeezing every few hours at first, and gradually more rapidly, until it is contracting more than once a minute at delivery. Physicians once ascribed the cause of most premature labor to womanly stress (the misogynist term "hysteria" is derived from the Greek *hysterikos*, or uterus), but modern obstetricians understand that early contractions are often a sign that something is wrong with the fetus, such as infection. Since the lungs are the critical determinant of when a baby is ready to be born, obstetricians are frequently hesitant to deliver a baby two months early.

Justine's doctors had tried to convince her uterus to relax, to take its time, a process of negotiation first begun with a shot of terbutaline under the skin, which sometimes places the uterus back into hibernation until the nine months are up. That didn't work. Soon afterward, both magnesium and terbutaline were administered intravenously, also without appreciable effect. It appeared that no amount of chemical persuasion was going to work on Justine's uterus. Then there was a complication. Over the past two hours, monitors placed on Justine's abdomen had indicated that the twins' heart rates were periodically decreasing, a sign that could mean worsening infection or a lack of oxygen. The children were no longer safe in Justine's uterus. Whereas previously the obstetricians tried to postpone delivery as long as possible, it now became imperative to deliver the babies quickly. The fastest way to get them out was by performing a cesarean section.

I glanced back to the center of the room and still couldn't see Justine's face. Her husband, an Irish-American man of about thirty named Paul, sat on a stool at the head of the operating table and held Justine's hand, which extended into my field of view. I walked a few paces over to gain some connection to the woman whose large abdomen was lit majestically in the center of the suite by high-intensity lamps. Paul was whispering continuously into his wife's ear, as tears rolled down her face. Justine lay on her back on a table in the middle of the operating room, saying over and over, "They're not ready. They're not ready. I'm not ready." Monitors at the head of the table indicated her heart rate, respiratory rate, and blood oxygen content. Numb from a spinal anesthesia, Justine's belly was painted a dark brown with an antiseptic. A long horizontal incision had been made.

I walked again to the warming table where Adam would be brought, and returned to the tackle box. We were ready to reel Adam into the world of the living. Mary, the triage nurse, hooked up the oxygen supply to the wall source, obtained warming blankets, and set the warming table temperature high, slightly over one hundred degrees. One of the biggest problems with newborns is that they can cool down rapidly since they are born wet. "Got the pipe?" she asked, referring to the endotracheal tube I had picked out. "Yup," I answered. "You better get an extra one, one size up," she advised smoothly, her voice just above the hiss of oxygen emanating from the tubes she connected. I liked Mary, with her no-nonsense attitude, and was lucky to have her confidence. NICU nurses are famously distrustful of green residents like myself. Once, Mary told me, the nurses had thrown a newborn baby to an intern they didn't like. The intern screamed, fell to the floor to break the baby's fall, and only then realized the "baby" was actually a plastic doll.

The obstetricians were still a few moments away from opening the uterus and delivering Adam, so I introduced myself to Paul and Justine. "Hi, I'm Dr. Sanghavi. We're going to take care of your little ones." I always called an unborn child "your little one" since one was never sure what sex the kid would be. I cautioned, "Since they're being born early, they probably won't be able to breathe well on their own, and we'll have to put a tube down their throats and into their lungs to help them breathe. You'll be able to see them and just maybe touch them, and then we'll have to take them upstairs." Paul swallowed, looked blankly at me, and nodded. Justine didn't say anything. I opened my mouth to offer additional words of encouragement, but the obstetricians had begun to incise the uterus. I scooted back to the warmer and joined Mary.

Suddenly, clear fluid fountained from Justine's abdomen. The obstetricians had broken her water and suctioned the fluid with vacuum-powered hoses that extended to receptacles several yards away. The hoses writhed as fluid rushed through them. I could see Adam's head, the size of a large orange, poking through the uterus, the body still hidden. Quickly, the obstetrician harvested the child, literally reaping him from the uterus by pulling him out by his head. With another rapid movement, he severed the umbilical cord, and in that motion the obstetrician's responsibility for Adam's life ended.

In the same motion, my responsibility began. Like a quarter-back, the obstetrician handed off Adam to the scrub nurse, who ran the newborn over to the warming table, and deposited him in front of me. Touchdown, I thought. Adam, covered by blood and amniotic fluid, didn't move at all, didn't breathe. He just lay there, blue as the sea. "It's a boy!" I heard one of the nurses say to Justine.

Usually, babies cry when they're delivered; the first breath heralds a stunning transformation in the lungs, which are full of amniotic fluid in utero. A baby doesn't need to breathe in the womb, since the mother's blood carries oxygen to the baby through the placenta, a sort of life-support organ attached to the uterus. During birth, the mother's support abruptly ends, and the child must breathe on his or her own, with lungs that have never been used. Pushed through the narrow birth canal, the child is squeezed and stressed so much that a surge of adrenaline is released, a baby's first natural high. The hormones jolt the baby's nervous system, and the result is an overwhelming neonatal arousal, a sentinel orgasm, expressed in the only way that the child can express feeling: by crying. The slap delivered to newborn buttocks on television shows is an unnecessary drama.

The baby's cry is really a first breath, a motion that unfurls the newborn lungs like sails. Billowing in the chest, the lungs suddenly begin to receive blood from the heart (which previously bypassed the lungs through a special blood vessel). At the warming table a pediatrician sees a sudden ripening of the baby; the brilliant blue of the baby's skin turns to a pink glow within seconds. "He's a rose," Mary would purr contentedly when we presided over a healthy delivery.

But Mary didn't say anything when Adam came to us. She roughly dried him with the towels, and I rubbed his back trying to stimulate an adrenaline surge, since cesarean deliveries don't produce as much squeezing and stress to provoke adrenaline as do vaginal deliveries. In my mind's eye, I remembered from boyhood summers in New Jersey trying to start the lawnmower for the first time of the season, pulling and pulling the starter cord, while the machine sputtered with false starts, until finally it began turning over. But ten seconds passed, and Adam just lay there on his back, not breathing.

"Tube him," said a voice behind me.

It was Sanjiv Khanna, the supervising neonatologist, who was watching over my shoulder. Sanjiv knew that time was critical to a newborn infant; every second we waited was another second that Adam's brain was starving for oxygen. Delay could mean a lifetime of cerebral palsy or brain damage for Adam. Adam had failed to breathe on his own, and it was our turn to take over.

Intubation, or the placement of a breathing tube into the windpipe, is the first step in a critically ill newborn's resuscitation. It's a very difficult procedure. Everything about a premature baby is small, including the windpipe, and getting the tube in the right place takes practice. It's something like defusing a bomb; there's limited time to succeed, and if you fail, someone dies.

"*Now,*" insisted Sanjiv.

Adam was lying on his back, with his head tilted toward me. I took the laryngoscope, a blunt metal blade with a lighted bulb on its tip, inserted it deep into Adam's mouth, and pulled toward the ceiling. Adam didn't gag or cough. His tongue was lifted and I saw into his throat. A tiny curve of skin the size and shape of a fingernail clipping, the epiglottis, stood guard at the base of the tongue. Every time food is swallowed, the epiglottis slaps up to cover the entrance to the trachea, blocking any food from getting into the lungs. Once in a great while, though, it fails, leading to choking. Although it seems strange to have the mouth and nose share a common passageway, it makes sense when one has a stuffy nose. If the mouth didn't also have a passageway to the lungs, a person would suffocate.

Holding the laryngoscope in my left hand, I took the 2.5 French tube in my right, and inserted it into Adam's mouth. I worked the tip toward the epiglottis and pushed the tube into the opening just below it. Two sail-like folds became visible in the opening; they were the vocal cords. I felt Sanjiv move forward impatiently, ready to take over from me. Though my hands were shaking a bit, I finally worked the tip of the tube past the cords. It all took about six seconds. Adam was tubed. I removed the laryngoscope, and Mary took over. Though the room was cold, I reached up to wipe sweat from my forehead.

Mary attached a rubber bag to the end of the tube. This bag in turn is connected by a second tube to an oxygen pump. The rubber bag served as Adam's lungs. Mary squeezed and released the bag vigorously about once every two seconds, forcing oxygen from the bag into Adam. At the same time, Sanjiv listened to Adam's heart and lungs with his stethoscope. The biggest mistake I could have made was to insert the tube into the esophagus instead of the trachea, which would simply lead to oxygen being pumped into Adam's belly. But Sanjiv gave me a thumbs up; he heard air move in the lungs.

"Heart rate's up," he called, meaning that Adam's heart was beating faster, a sign that oxygen was reaching his body. "And there's condensation in the tube. But I don't hear air on the left side of the chest."

The trachea branches into two segments, or mainstem bronchi: one that enters the right lung and one that enters the left. Frequently, a small child who chokes on a peanut or piece of popcorn—foods not recommended by the American Academy of Pediatrics for any toddler—has lodged the item in the right mainstem bronchus since it has a more favorable angle of entry from the trachea. Similarly, I had inserted the tube too far into Adam's lungs, directly into his right mainstem. That's why Sanjiv couldn't hear any air in Adam's left lung; only the right was getting oxygen.

"Pull back the tube," Sanjiv said to me, in the somewhat understated but urgent tone of a flight instructor telling a novice pilot to "pull back on the stick" to avoid a crash landing. I retracted the tube about one centimeter so that both mainstems received oxygen, and Sanjiv listened again to Adam's chest and smiled. "Equal breath sounds," he said.

Mary beamed as Adam's skin turned pink. "He's a rose," she concluded.

The baby's father, Paul, accompanied Mary and me from the operating room to the NICU. On the elevator, as Mary squeezed the bag giving oxygen and life to Adam, Paul told me in an emotional voice about how hard he and Justine had tried for children, and about visits to various fertility experts. To have children was the most powerful longing he had ever felt, Paul said. Justine had gotten pregnant by artificial insemination after four years of attempts. "It's a goddamn miracle," he said hoarsely, gazing at his child. We saw things so differently, I thought. I was fixated on the warmer that kept Adam's body temperature up, the oxygen bag that inflated his lungs, and the tones of his heart through my stethoscope. Paul didn't see a critically ill child; he looked at a heaven-sent gift, a perfect newborn son whom he would one day teach to eat with a spoon, to throw a ball, and to tie a shoe.

Medical knowledge can be a mixed blessing. Physicians develop an enormous ability to deconstruct complex biological systems. By reducing a person to his components, they can evaluate and treat many problems. A doctor may ask, "Are you tired? Let's take you apart: we'll check your blood for anemia, your lungs for hypoxia, your endocrine system for hypothyroidism, your heart for inflammation," and so on. We develop a taste for pathology, a powerful satisfaction at finding something wrong after a careful search. Doctors lose some of their appreciation for health; it makes us feel useless. After all, if Adam had been an entirely normal child, my presence would have been irrelevant.

With maturity, a physician realizes that good health in a patient is far more satisfying. Many years ago, the son of an artist named Sigmund Abeles was born prematurely at the Brigham NICU. Day after day, Abeles sat at his son's bedside and drew charcoal sketches of him, complete with the maze of surrounding medical machines. As the days went by, fewer and fewer tubes and probes remained, until one day Abeles drew only his son. Through drawing, he extracted his son from the morass of medical equipment around him. Reproductions of Abeles's drawings hang in the NICU today, reminders to us that newborn children are emerging human spirits.

Looking at the form in the clear plastic incubator, I struggled to connect with the small mass of flesh called Adam. Health isn't something for physicians to fear, I thought, but an invitation to connect with others. The key is to stop viewing ourselves as providers and children like Adam as clients. After all, it wasn't every day you get to witness a miracle like Paul and Justine's little child. I reached out a hand to Paul's shoulder, which trembled with emotion. His eyes met mine, and we didn't need to say anything.

Adam was brought to the NICU and "booked." Electrical wires were taped to his chest to follow his heart rate and breathing, his breathing tube was hooked to a mechanical ventilator, and intra-venous catheters were inserted into his veins. Instead of showing clear, dark lungs, a chest X ray showed them filled with fine, dusty shadows. This was the hallmark of premature lungs, and the dusty shadows were going to be a problem. Adam's twin, a little girl named Evelyn, was on a warmer next to him. A second resident had man-aged her in the delivery room. She too had shadows on her X ray.

The shadows indicated the presence of thousands of small, balloon-like areas called alveoli. In the lungs, the mainstem bronchi subdivide into smaller and smaller branches, which end in the alve-oli, the cul-de-sacs of the pulmonary neighborhood. In healthy full-term infants, the alveoli are filled with air, but in Adam's and Evelyn's lungs they remained collapsed, giving their X rays a hazy appearance.

There is a curious property of lungs I unknowingly demonstrated as a child blowing up balloons for my sister's birthday parties. I'd take a balloon, stretch it out to limber it up, and blow into it. Nothing would happen. I'd take a deeper breath, and blow harder. A small, temporary inflation resulted, which summarily deflated. Thoroughly frustrated, I then took my mightiest breath and blew with every muscle in my thorax. The balloon finally submitted and accepted the air. Subsequent breaths to complete the inflation were far easier—the process was analogous to loosening a jar's lid, where the hardest part is the first twist.

Adam's lungs were just like those birthday balloons: high pres-sures were required to pop open the alveoli for the first time. Once open, they'd require far less effort to keep them inflated. Since most of Adam's alveoli were closed, we also were forced to pump high concentrations of oxygen into his lungs to keep him from suffocat-ing. But oxygen in pure form at high pressure is a surprisingly deadly substance. The same attribute that makes oxygen a key bio-logical necessity—its startling ability to react with organic com-pounds—allows it to harm healthy areas of the lungs if breathed for long at the concentrations we were using. Adam's appetite for oxygen would be a self-destructive gluttony unless we could inflate his lungs more easily.

Adam was one of about 20,000 to 30,000 infants who are born yearly in the United States with immature lungs, or "respiratory distress syndrome." Until 1959, no one knew why these newborns couldn't breathe properly, and many of them died. Mary Ellen Avery, a pediatrician at Children's Hospital in Boston, discovered that year that many premature babies lack a key compound called surfactant, a slippery, soapy substance that makes it easier for the lungs to inflate. No one was able to use this knowledge to help newborns until 1972, when G. C. Liggins and R. N. Howie discovered that steroids injected into mothers undergoing premature labor caused their unborn fetuses to produce surfactant. Unfortunately, this wasn't a perfect solution; despite receiving steroids many mothers still delivered newborns with respiratory distress syndrome.

Adam was one of them. We could have proven this by taking a half teaspoon of Justine's amniotic fluid, mixing it with an equal volume of grain alcohol in a tube, and shaking it up. No bubbles would have appeared, signifying a lack of surfactant. Amniotic fluid is simply a baby's urine and is a valuable indicator of a baby's surfactant level since it is breathed in and out of the lungs in utero. It is critical in expanding the lungs and causing them to develop. In some congenital kidney diseases where a fetus cannot make amniotic fluid, the lungs never develop, leading to a fatal condition called Potter's syndrome.

In 1980, a group of Japanese pediatricians led by T. Fujiwara successfully took surfactant purified from cow lungs and administered it to a premature baby. Since then, surfactant (or "surf," as we called it in the NICU) has become a key reason that almost all premature babies of Adam's gestational age are able to survive.

Dottie Upshaw, the respiratory therapist, flicked back her short red hair. "Are we gonna surf, or what?" she drawled, as she adjusted Adam's ventilator. Dottie loved lung physiology, and often said things like "I'll need to up the delta P on the oscillator a bit, since the hypercarbia's a problem, but don't worry, the MAP is only 18 torr, and I don't think elastic compliance is a problem." I knew better than to question a woman like that. "Let's do it," I agreed.

Dottie showed me a bottle containing a tablespoon of milky fluid, and pulled it into a syringe. "Here, feel a drop," she said, and dribbled a little on my fingers. It was the most slippery material I'd ever experienced; I could hardly bring my fingers together before they slipped apart. The substance seemed to completely dispel friction. "That's surfactant," Dottie said proudly. "And that drop probably costs ten dollars. That vial costs over one thousand dollars, so let's be sure not to drop it."

We approached Adam's unit and watched the ventilator give him breaths, at pressures almost twice what is required by an adult. Remarkably, Adam's chest barely expanded; he was just like one of my sister's birthday balloons. Listening to his chest with my stethoscope, I heard the crackling, popping noises of immature lungs. Sanjiv called the noise "the washing machine in Adam's chest."

Dottie emptied the syringe of surfactant directly into Adam's breathing tube. Almost immediately, Adam's chest began rising like a loaf of bread. The surfactant invaded Adam's collapsed alveoli, which began popping open like cell doors in a jailbreak. Adam's lungs were inflating, free at last. The following day, the ventilator was removed and Adam took his first breath by himself. He even yawned once. Though it was several weeks before Adam and his sibling left the NICU—they still needed to develop better temperature-regulation and eating skills, typical problems in premature infants—the rest of their NICU days were quiet ones.

I had many conversations with Justine and Paul over this time, updating them regularly on the twins' progress. They never stopped mentioning the "breathing medicine" that let their new children survive. "You could say I was obsessed with the idea of having kids," Justine once confessed. "It's all I ever thought about. And now I can move on. I feel like a weight's been lifted off me." It seemed that Adam and Evelyn weren't the only ones whose chests were freed.

Bobby Aire, a five-year-old, had developed a curious reflex: he took deep, sighing breaths whenever a doctor approached with a stethoscope. On the day we met, I placed the bell of my stethoscope just below his shoulder blade. Between breaths, Bobby sang various cartoon theme songs. The words sounded muffled, as if sung through an empty tunnel.

A small child, Bobby often had trouble keeping up with his first-grade classmates. Over the past few weeks, he had found it harder to make it to first base during kickball games and sat out of many gym classes from shortness of breath. The decline came insidiously.

As I lowered the stethoscope farther down Bobby's back, his songs suddenly became clear and comprehensible, as if sung directly in my ear. A portion of his lung was filled with fluid, which conducts higher-frequency sounds better than air. The fluid was pus, the putrid, yellow stuff the immune system produces to kill bacterial invaders. Bobby had pneumonia, and this was his third hospitalization in as many years.

Getting pneumonia even once is not easy. Owing to the lungs' proximity to one of the most polluted spaces of the body—the nose and mouth—they possess formidable defenses against invasion. A bacterium inhaled into the nose can quickly be expelled by a sneeze, or trapped in the mucus that coats the membranes behind the nose, then swept into the stomach and destroyed by hydrochloric acid. If the microorganism is fortunate enough to be inhaled into the trachea, it is likely captured in the mucus that lines the bronchi. Each cell that makes up the bronchus has over two hundred cilia, or tiny hairs, that whip one thousand times per minute away from the direction of airflow. These microscopic oars push invaders trapped in the tenacious mucus and expel them out of the trachea and into the esophagus. In short order, the invaders are digested.

Once in a while a microbe gets sneezed or coughed in an airborne particle so small that one hundred of them laid side by side would be as wide as the period at the end of this sentence. Such a particle can remain suspended in a room's atmosphere for a long time. When inhaled, it occasionally makes it past all the defenses of the victim's lung, and lands in the smallest airways, the alveoli. There, patrolling sentries called alveolar macrophages usually recognize these intruders, engulf them, and dismantle them with destructive enzymes.

Despite all of these defenses, some microbes do successfully infect the lungs of children. The most common, *Streptococcus pneumoniae*, enter alveoli, avoid capture by macrophages via a camouflaged coating, and begin to multiply. After a short time, the immune system alerts to the intruders and begins a scorched-earth attack, bombing the infected areas of the lung with pus. In response, a child develops fever and difficulty breathing as the lungs fill with pus. Pneumonia, the inflammation of the lung's cellular structure, begins.

As his mother looked on, amused, Bobby completed his repertoire of cartoon jingles and moved on to the alphabet song. Typically, children with pneumonia have high fevers and deep, hacking coughs. Sometimes, they have only vomiting or severe abdominal pain. Once, when I was a second-year resident, one child even underwent a misguided appendectomy before his doctors realized he had pneumonia.

Bobby was an unusual patient because he repeatedly acquired infections. There are many reasons a child can have recurrent pneumonias. Bobby could have a malfunctioning immune system from HIV infection or any of a host of genetic problems, like severe combined immunodeficiency or the so-called bubble boy syndrome. He could have Kartagener's syndrome, where the hairs that line the bronchi are missing. (Oddly, these patients also have bodies that are mirror images of normal ones: their hearts and spleens are on the right side and their livers and stomachs on the left.) Bobby, though, had a much more common problem.

"I have sixty-five roses," volunteered Bobby. Many children use an alternative vocabulary for complex disease names. Hence, some say "smiling mighty Jesus" in place of spinal meningitis, or "Luke and Leia" instead of leukemia, or Bobby's phrase, "sixty-five roses," instead of the reason he had already been admitted three times for pneumonia: cystic fibrosis, or CF.

The term *cystic fibrosis* describes the chest X rays of patients like Bobby. Instead of clean, dark areas, the lung fields develop multiple bubblelike sacs, or cysts, giving the lung the appearance of Swiss cheese. These cysts are stiff with scarring, or fibrosis. The disease affects one in twenty-five hundred white Americans, about five to twenty times more often than it strikes nonwhites. Only about a quarter of these patients survives to adulthood, and fewer than one in ten lives past the age of thirty.

In 1990, an international collaboration among biochemists discovered the cause of cystic fibrosis, the most common fatal genetic disease of white Americans. In patients with CF, a single component of the cell's outer covering, or membrane, doesn't move salt as well as it should. This inadequate regulation of salt molecules is especially pronounced in the lungs, where it interferes with the immune system and ultimately causes recurrent infections. Patients with CF have continuous pneumonia, and are admitted to the hospital every few months for antibiotic treatment. One of my patients said cystic fibrosis was like "peanut butter in your lungs, and no matter how hard you cough, it never moves."

Periodically, these infections with bacteria possessing salacious names like *Pseudomonas aeroginosa* and *Burkholderia cepacia* would lead to too much peanut butter–like material in the lungs. Bobby felt increasingly short of breath, and his mother would know it was time for a "tune-up." That's when he came to the hospital. These admissions typically lasted a few weeks. During this time, his veins were filled with a cornucopia of antibiotics like aztreonam, piperacillin, tazobactam, tobramycin, trimethoprim, sulfamethoxasole, and ciprofloxicin. This antimicrobial onslaught would obliterate pneumonia in any other person, but in CF patients like Bobby, it merely loosened the peanut butter slightly.

Twice a day, a physical therapist—typically a well-muscled individual—pounded Bobby's back with a medley of blows. From outside the room, I heard clomping sounds reminiscent of a team of horses on asphalt. This was chest physiotherapy, a technique for further loosening the peanut butter. From time to time, the therapist paused, and Bobby coughed thick, foul secretions into a pail at his bedside. He usually felt better after these purgative sessions. Day after day, he reclaimed small areas of his lungs, adding a few extra teaspoons of space for air instead of the peanut butter. "Gross, huh?" he said once, proudly showing off his bucket of mucus.

These hospitalizations offer improvement for only a few months, until the pneumonia progresses enough that another tune-up is necessary. Over the years, Bobby's deterioration was documented exquisitely. Pulmonary function tests, or PFTs, are measured by blowing as hard as possible into a long tube that looks like a vacuum cleaner hose. One's lung volume is immediately displayed on a computer screen, and the number essentially tells a patient how long he has to live. The more fibrosis you have, the lower your numbers. In CF, they unrelentingly get worse year after year, and Bobby's were no exception. It's a terrifying prospect for many children. Bobby's friends, Sarah and Annie Ramsey, were mischievous eight-year-old twins with CF who could handle almost any procedure, including painful arterial blood tests, without flinching. But the simple, painless pulmonary function test was so daunting that the girls literally had to be dragged to the machine. They knew what the numbers meant, and Sarah's numbers were worsening much faster than Annie's. With each PFT session, the twins were reminded that Sarah would likely die first.

At the age of five, the only indication that Bobby wasn't like other boys was his slightly small stature, and his yearly admissions to the hospital for treatment of pneumonia. Though the east wing of the tenth floor of the hospital was devoted to patients with Bobby's illness, Bobby's mother refused to allow him to be treated there and insisted on another wing. "I don't want Bobby to see *them*," she said. "He already knows he's different."

Like many parents, Bobby's mother struggled to preserve her son's innocence from the realities of his illness. Though he sang songs without a care, his lungs were inexorably deteriorating year after year. The care of people with cystic fibrosis introduced me to one of life's tragic disappointments: stories without proper endings. Someday, perhaps even in a few years, Bobby's lungs would be just like Peter West's.

Peter West was a forty-year-old mechanic whom I cared for as a second-year resident. (Though Children's is a pediatric facility, many patients with CF continue to receive their care at our hospital.) The first time we met, I had just sent several patient reports from my work terminal to the printer located in the nurse's station and had walked over to retrieve them. There I came across a squat gray-haired man with leathery hands, tinkering with the air vent on the printer. I looked closer, interested, and saw he had created a fingernail-sized fan out of paper, and hooked it to the exhaust vent of the printer. The fan spun merrily, and Peter concentrated on it with an amused expression.

He turned his face to me. "I'm Peter," he began, and I immediately noticed his T-shirt. The shirt was covered with a graph depicting the results of his lung function tests over time. "The Rise and Fall of Peter West," read the title above the graph. I scrutinized the most recent point on the graph, from a month earlier. His total lung capacity was less than a third of normal, a level almost incompatible with living.

We started talking. "I'm in for a tune-up, the usual every few months. You one of the new docs?" "Yes," I answered. "Nice to see you," he said, turning his attention back to the printer.

Not one for denial, Peter wore his lungs on his sleeve, displaying his results on his T-shirt. As the days went by, Peter intrigued me more and more. How was he able to deal with the pressure of his condition? To get to know him better, I visited him often in the evenings. Because the hospital wing was primarily used to care for CF patients, Peter had gotten to know many other adults and children with CF. He was rarely alone, since others would drop by his room to gossip. I heard a variety of news about the wing's residents: Lou had once left the hospital in the middle of one of his tune-ups to go drinking at a bar, and been arrested for fighting. Cherry was getting a divorce. Amanda was going to college to study architecture.

One night, just before Peter turned in for the evening, he and I were alone. He looked uncharacteristically weary as he prepared to attach a breathing mask to his face so he wouldn't suffocate overnight. He'd had to wear this apparatus for the past few months, since he had become a "carbon dioxide retainer." Generally, when a person holds his breath, an uncomfortable sensation creeps into the chest, until his entire being crackles with the unbearable need to breathe. This isn't because the person is running out of oxygen; on the contrary, lungs hold enough oxygen to last several minutes without exhaling and inhaling. The nemesis is carbon dioxide, which builds up quickly when you don't breathe. The brain finds carbon dioxide utterly intolerable and urges exhalation within seconds of breath holding. Thus, the feeling of suffocation is the feeling of carbon dioxide in the brain.

This is all for good reason; if deprived of oxygen for even minutes, the brain would die. Increasing levels of carbon dioxide serve as an early warning mechanism that something bad is afoot. Peter's lungs, though, were so scarred that his carbon dioxide levels were always high. Like a battered spouse who comes to expect her abuse, Peter's brain simply accepted the high levels of carbon dioxide, especially while he was sleeping. Without a mask, Peter's levels would rise very high. At these levels, carbon dioxide has an insidious effect on the brain, causing it gradually to slip into an oblivious "carbon dioxide narcosis." Without breathing assistance, Peter's brain would happily tolerate the peace of carbon dioxide narcosis and neglect breathing completely. He would pass away without a care.

Peter fingered the mask idly and whispered, "Sometimes dying doesn't seem so bad." He said he felt so trapped in his body, so very tired. Last night he'd dreamed he was swimming underwater, without breathing. He looked to his sides and saw gills. He was free of a world where lungs mattered, or even existed. That was the only way to make it all better: forgetting lungs altogether.

As a patient with CF, Peter was accustomed to disappointment. Foremost was the failed promise of gene therapy. Currently, the medical literature of CF is littered with articles about adenoviruses, liposomal DNA delivery, vectors, and other methods of repairing the genes of patients like Peter. Unfortunately, fixing the salt channel gene is turning out to be much harder than thought. Like that of the gene for sickle cell anemia (known for almost fifty years), the knowledge of the CF gene has not found therapeutic use. Perhaps some patients feel better knowing that like the defective hemoglobin in sickle cell anemia, which protects against malaria, the faulty channel of CF may have protected generations of people from *Salmonella* infections. But this seems a rather abstract comfort.

Most patients with CF have an erroneous single nucleotide—out of three billion—coding for the 508th amino acid of the cystic fibrosis trans-membrane receptor. The tantalizing simplicity of this single error fires the dreams of gene therapists worldwide. It is just a few molecules, after all. But a cure isn't coming soon enough for

Peter; the technology doesn't yet exist. Death from cystic fibrosis is his destiny. As in a sonnet, he possesses freedom to write some verse in his life, but overall structure is predetermined.

Peter remembered the day the gene was discovered. "I breathed a little easier that day," he said. I asked him if he thought he had been offered a false hope. He smiled. "The thing is, 'false hope' is an oxymoron. I always appreciate extra hope." Peter placed the mask over his face, looking like a scuba diver ready to submerge. "I like sleeping," he said, "since I've been having nice dreams lately." He closed his eyes, and his breathing slowed. As Peter stopped breathing deeply, his ventilator began dispensing breaths. The soft blowing sounds reminded me of ocean waves lapping at shore, an image of renewal.

Somewhat at peace, I walked over to the intensive care unit to visit Joannie Simpson, another resident. Though my ward was quiet, I wasn't ready to go to bed yet. I knew Joannie would be up; an intensive care unit resident rarely had time to sleep.

She was managing a full house of patients, but one stood out. Angelina Todd, a fifteen-year-old with CF, had suffered a severe lung bleed, an uncommon complication of scarred lungs. She was sedated and had a breathing tube down her throat. Pink froth bubbled in the tube. Angelina was so emaciated that her skin looked like a thin sheet placed over a skeleton. She was attached to machines from head to toe, with invasive catheters and tubes in every orifice. Her body had no secrets. Every vital parameter was measured and displayed on computer screens. This was cystic fibrosis at its most devastating. Angelina was dying publicly, and Bobby and Peter would probably die the same way someday.

The breathing machine supporting Angelina made a high-pitched noise. A nurse detached the machine, rinsed Angelina's breathing tube with saline, and suctioned out clots of blood. He reattached the tube, and the machine ceased its alarms. Because Angelina was alone (her family was driving in to see her), I sat at her bedside and watched the machine breathe for her. After five minutes, I couldn't take it anymore. I was so disturbed by the hopelessness of CF that I began to wheeze slightly, and my breathing became labored. I pulled my inhaler out of my lab coat and blasted a puff of albuterol into my lungs. The wheezing disappeared, but the pressure of Bobby and Peter and Angelina's tragedies remained.

Wheezing is the breathless, low whistle made by air exhaled through constricted airways deep in the lungs. It is uncomfortable; one can reproduce the sensation by running up several flights of stairs and then breathing through a soft-drink straw. Many things cause wheezing, including acid indigestion, heart failure, and even a small object like a raisin aspirated into the lung. But by far the most common reason for wheezing, and the reason that almost one-tenth of all children wheeze at some time, is asthma.

Working in the emergency room early one morning, I saw Shakeera Jordan, a nine-year-old girl who was wheezing. "I woke up last night and," she panted, "I couldn't breathe. My mother," she panted, "gave me a treatment, but it didn't"—she paused again—"help." Shakeera's mother, Cheryl, lived in a tenement on the South Side of Boston. She had been through all of this before; her daughter had acute attacks requiring hospitalization every few months. Cheryl looked exhausted and frustrated. "I got rid of the cat, ripped up the carpets, and bought special sheets for her bed. I did everything I was supposed to. How come she's still sick all the time?" she demanded.

I didn't know. Though common, asthma is a perplexing condition. Asthmatics can be prompted to wheeze by a large variety of exposures, including wood shavings, cold air, carpeting, laundry detergents, dusty pillows or stuffed animals, ozone, cockroaches, mold, stress, cats, medications, cold viruses, food preservatives or colors, aspirin, or scores of other things. For a child like Shakeera, who had no easily identifiable trigger, parents are forced to turn their dwellings upside down for a cause. Worse, these changes frequently have no beneficial effect.

Shakeera's mother told me a visiting nurse had inspected her home, noting cockroach infestation, dusty carpeting, and a radiator leak that allowed mold to grow on several walls. Shakeera's mother had done what she could, but her landlord had not yet fixed the pipes or paid for extermination. Her pediatrician had written a letter to the city housing authority, and she had called the mayor's housing hotline, but nothing had happened. This was a typical theme. In a city with less than 1 percent housing vacancy and minimal low-income housing in safe areas, tenants are extremely unwilling to upset landlords. So children like Shakeera continue to wheeze, trapped in housing with moldy walls.

Shakeera was in a fair amount of respiratory distress now. "Let's get her some nebulizer treatments," I said to a circulating nurse. We placed a small plastic mask over Shakeera's mouth and nose, and attached a salt shaker–sized chamber to the bottom of the mask. Into the salt shaker, or reservoir, we placed ten drops of a clear solution, and added a half teaspoon of salt water. We were almost ready. Finally, we ran a clear plastic tube from the reservoir to an oxygen pump, and turned on the pump. The oxygen atomized, or "nebulized," the liquid in the reservoir, and a fine mist collected in Shakeera's mask. She breathed it hungrily.

The clear solution was magic as far as I was concerned. As a child, I had struggled to keep up in school gym class, felt especially short of breath on cold days, and often woke up coughing at night. Though I later had my first acute asthma attack in India, I was not diagnosed until I returned to the United States. In my physician's office that day, I had received the same treatment I was now giving Shakeera. I remember taking deep breaths, aware that air was entering areas of lung I never knew existed. The relief was instantaneous. I felt liberated; not only could I breathe, but I realized that my exercise limitation wasn't my own fault. The next day, after taking two puffs of the same medicine from a handheld inhaler, I ran a mile for the first time in my life.

The fundamental problem in asthma is that the lungs are too twitchy. When an offending trigger—for example, house dust (which is actually fecal waste from mites)—enters the lungs, tiny muscle fibers around the airways tighten up. Nobody knows why. This constriction makes it exceedingly difficult to move air; hence, the wheezing sound. The medication in the clear solution, albuterol, forces these muscles to relax. The uterus has many of the same types of muscles. Drugs related to albuterol are often used to relax the uterus, and stop premature labor.

Shakeera inhaled the first dose of albuterol in about twenty minutes, but she continued to breathe fast and uncomfortably. Her nurse and I refilled her reservoir, and the mist appeared again. Shakeera refused to answer questions now; this wasted too much of her precious air. She sat with her hands hooked to the chair, using them as supports while she strained for air. Every time she inhaled, the skin over her collarbone and neck was sucked in, indicating the tremendous inhalation pressure she was using. She was working hard.

A third dose was required. Shakeera had been breathing the mist for almost an hour, without substantially improving. Following a protocol for asthmatic children in distress, I ordered a tablespoon of a pink liquid called methylprednisolone. This is a type of steroid, a hormone made from cholesterol. Along with the muscular jumpiness, asthmatic lungs also have significant swelling and inflammation. Certain steroids, like the pink liquid, have potent anti-inflammatory properties and have been shown to lessen wheezing. Unfortunately, the taste is so vile that children invariably spit it up. To her credit Shakeera didn't, although she made an ugly face while swallowing.

Cheryl was increasingly agitated. "Why isn't Shakeera getting better? She looks worse." She was right. Shakeera looked awfully tired, almost like she was going to give up soon. Asthma is a war of attrition; the lung constriction almost always lets up after some time, usually dramatically. But until then, you had to fight it. If Shakeera was getting fatigued now, that was ominous.

When taking care of a child like Shakeera who seems to be quite ill, a pediatrician comes to a critical juncture. Do you continue the standard therapy and hope the child improves? Or do you activate the next level of care? That means calling the intensive care unit, putting in invasive intravenous lines, getting X rays, and generally sounding an alarm. False alarms are a serious nuisance, potentially removing people from other patients.

I spoke to Dr. Barker, the attending physician in the emergency room. He examined Shakeera, and agreed she looked ill. "You should get a gas," he advised, "and run it by the intensive care unit."

Dr. Barker meant that I needed to take a blood sample from Shakeera's artery and see whether it had become acidic. Acid blood was a sign that Shakeera was retaining carbon dioxide, just like Peter West. However, unlike Peter, Shakeera wasn't used to this condition. If her blood was acidic, she was feeling suffocated, like someone holding her breath. Her best attempts to breathe harder and faster would be failing. That would mean she was physically incapable of generating enough power to fill her lungs. If that were the case, she'd need intensive care.

Arterial blood samples are much more painful than simple blood tests, because arteries have more sensitive nerves around them. Shakeera wasn't going to like this, and might move her hand when I inserted the needle. Thankfully, Eric was working today.

Eric is a "holder," a clinical assistant who works in the emergency room, a specialist in restraining children during painful procedures. Holding was a martial art of sorts, since a holder had to prevent a child's movement without inflicting injury. Good holders were crucial for procedures such as suturing facial lacerations, spinal taps, and blood tests. They were needed even when we used local anesthesia; for many children, fear is more of a problem than pain. Eric put his whole body into holding children, but he was gentle. We often said that getting a successful blood test in one stick or clear fluid from a spinal tap was mostly the result of a good holder, rather than a skilled physician.

"Shakeera, we're going to do a blood test," I said. "I'll numb it up so it only pinches a little. Lie down for a minute." She nodded. Her mother stroked the child's face. Eric stood next to Shakeera, placed his right hand under her elbow to extend her arm, and gripped her palm with his left hand. ("Always control a child's joints, and they won't move," he once told me.) I took the thinnest needle we had, pushed it through the skin on the wrist, and injected a few drops of lidocaine, a local anesthetic. Shakeera began to cry, but she didn't move. Next, I massaged the lidocaine into the wrist to numb the artery, and readied a second syringe. Shakeera stopped crying and listened to her mother tell a story. I felt for a pulse, found it, and inserted the needle. Bright red blood pulsed into the syringe. I removed the needle and put a bandage on the wrist. Eric relaxed his grip on Shakeera's arm and gave her a rabbit sticker as a reward.

I sent the sample to the lab and discussed the possible outcomes with Shakeera's mother. If the results of the blood test were discouraging, Shakeera would go to the intensive care unit. There, she would receive albuterol mist continuously. Because her breathing was so labored, the medicine may not be getting deep enough into her lungs. So we would also need to place an intravenous line and give her another medicine directly into her blood, which more reliably got to her lungs. She would also receive larger doses of steroids.

"What if all that fails?" Cheryl asked upon hearing all this.

Then, I explained, we could try a variety of other medicines. We could infuse magnesium into Shakeera to further relax her lungs (magnesium is another way to stop premature labor). Or she could breathe a mixture of helium and oxygen in her mask. Heliox, as this mixture is called, relies on the same principle known to children at birthday parties; inhaling helium makes you talk like a Munchkin. Helium is lighter than nitrogen, which usually makes up 70 percent of the air we breathe. Lighter gases move faster through narrow spaces. That's how helium causes your voice to be high, by moving faster through the vocal cords than nitrogen. If air could move faster out of Shakeera's lungs, she might breathe easier.

"What if that fails, too?" Cheryl persisted. Later, I learned that she had been waiting for new housing through the Section 8 federal program for almost a year. Her boyfriend was shot to death a few years ago. Her sister had been expelled from school. Cheryl was earning barely enough money to put food on the table. She expected worst-case scenarios.

Well, at that point we'd have to consider a breathing tube and general anesthesia, I said. But that rarely happens.

"Things that rarely happen, happen to me," Cheryl muttered. "I'm sick of it."

The blood gas results were returned about five minutes after I sent it. The blood was not acidic, but slightly alkaline. It was an encouraging result and I told Cheryl that Shakeera might not need intensive care. She grunted, evidently not persuaded that everything was all right. I asked the nurse to give Shakeera another dose of albuterol and told Cheryl I'd be back to see how her daughter responded. Ten minutes later, Shakeera's eyes had brightened somewhat and her breathing was improved. "We're supposed to study caterpillars in school," she said. "I'm missing it." Cheryl suppressed a smile at her child's words.

I admitted Shakeera from the emergency room to the pediatric ward, where she remained for two days. The social worker Louise Abode made innumerable phone calls on Shakeera and Cheryl's behalf to find better housing, places without moldy walls and cockroaches. Complaints against the landlord were filed. The family was placed on several housing lists, but nothing opened up before discharge. Shakeera returned home.

Like many illnesses affected by a child's environment, asthma is more prevalent (by 20 percent) among the urban poor than the general population. It is also more severe; the risk of mortality from asthma is three to nine times higher in these children. When exploring deep shafts, miners once used canaries as indicators of air quality, since these birds are very sensitive to toxic gases. If the canaries died, the miners knew that the air was contaminated. In poor living conditions, children are like the canaries. They're the first to suffer, giving us early clues about the livability of our cities. Emergency visits like Shakeera's are, unfortunately, more and more common. When a child like Shakeera comes to an emergency room, we're presented with a small opportunity not only to help her breathe more freely but to live more freely. As in Shakeera's case, we are often unsuccessful.

My own asthma is now well controlled, but I no longer take breathing for granted because of my father. Several years ago, his pulmonologist diagnosed him with asthma. The doctor was wrong. Recently my father was found to have a rare scarring condition of the lungs called idiopathic pulmonary fibrosis. (*Idiopathic* is a fancy medical way of saying, "Nobody knows what causes it.") A previously vigorous man, he went within a year from hiking mountain trails to barely making it to his bedroom wearing an oxygen tank.

When I visit my family at home in New Jersey, we make it a point to eat breakfast together. I watch my father as he eats his favorite Indian foods, like fried *chacoli*, dried *mumra*, and baked *khakhara*, washed down with a ginger-seasoned cup of *chai*. Eating is one of life's pleasures that he still can enjoy. But he sometimes laments his homebound state. Since he requires oxygen almost continually, he can no longer travel. Any trip, even to visit friends in nearby towns, requires days of planning to arrange enough oxygen tanks from his insurer. His world has gotten smaller.

After we eat, I lace up my running sneakers and step outside. Mornings are usually brisk, and the neighborhood is filled with sounds of cicadas and sparrows. My sneakers are sopping with dew by the time I walk through the grass to the road. Just before starting the run, I lift my albuterol inhaler to my mouth and take two satisfying puffs. I feel energized. I fill my lungs with the morning air and begin to run. I jog down to the old orchard, back to the middle school, and finally onto Mimosa Drive, a total of two miles.

My father greets me at the door when I return. Did you have a good time? he asks. Yes, I answer. "It must feel pretty good," he observes, "to be so free."

~ 2 ~

Heart

TALES WITH VARYING DEGREES OF CLOSURE

Joseph Abel was seventeen years old and clearly an athlete. His well-muscled torso, washboard abdomen, and powerful limbs were outlined by his bed linens in the intensive care unit. Indicating excellent aerobic condition, his heart beat regularly with a low pulse. Evan Fleur, the intensive care attending, once called Joseph's heart "magnificent."

But now Joseph was dead. Two days earlier he had been thrown from a motorcycle and suffered serious head trauma. He lacked all indicators of purposeful neurological activity, like spontaneous breathing, eye pupil reflexes, and response to touch. However, his body had suffered no significant injury. Though the mind and body are betrothed in life, no covenant requires their simultaneous death.

Joseph's heart continued to beat, his lungs continued to accept oxygen from the breathing machine, and his intestines continued to process the food placed in his stomach via a nasal tube. He even urinated intermittently since his kidneys worked fine. Joseph's body was like the string quartet aboard the *Titanic* as it sank; the oblivious musicians just continued playing.

After morning rounds I—a junior medical student at Johns Hopkins in Baltimore—was always the last to leave Joseph's room, since the team had a habit of leaving the room in order of rank. Perhaps his parents saw me as a more accessible member of the team, or at least one who shared their bewilderment at the changes in their family's life. They had trouble deciding whether to prolong the life of Joseph's body. "I know it doesn't make sense," his mother confessed to me one morning. "But maybe somewhere he can hear and feel me, don't you think?"

"I'm sure he can," I answered almost distractedly. Our eyes met, and for a moment I indeed believed that Joseph could hear his mother somewhere.

Joseph's parents wanted him to be an organ donor, Evan Fleur announced outside the room one day. A team of cardiac transplant surgeons was summoned from Pittsburgh to take his heart, or, in the parlance of transplant surgery, "harvest the organ." I find the term comforting; a harvest season is a time of joy, the reaping of the earth's bounty for nourishment.

Sometime in the afternoon, Joseph was wheeled to the operating room. About thirty minutes into the procedure, the surgeons cut a long incision into Joseph's chest, and sawed apart his rib cage to expose the beating heart.

It was a magnificent and terrible sight. Slightly larger than a softball, Joseph's heart alternately swelled and collapsed in an orderly top-to-bottom fashion, about once every second. It had done this without pause for the past seventeen years, hidden until today. The light from the overhead lamps now brightly illuminated the heart.

Five feet away, I could make out its anatomy. The surface was largely covered by glistening yellow fat, its normal coat. A few wormlike structures were also visible below that fat; these were the coronary arteries, the blood vessels that give oxygen to the heart.

Centuries earlier, blood was thought to have sloshed in a disorderly manner throughout the body, and the heart was considered a porous organ of no clear mechanical significance. William Harvey, a sixteenth-century Oxford anatomist, examined the blood vessels of almost eighty different animals, including dogs, fish, and man, and discovered an unusual property of veins. When he forced water through veins toward the heart, the water proceeded without resistance. However, when he tried to inject water in the opposite direction, it would not pass. Harvey discovered a principle clear to anyone who's played a reed instrument; you can produce results only by blowing air in one direction through the instrument's reed. Small valves similar to saxophone mouthpieces punctuate veins. Harvey realized that blood *circulates* in a single direction, and that the heart is a mechanical pump.

The human heart is composed of a right and left side. Blood returning to the heart from the body collects in the upper right chamber of the heart, called the right atrium. Passing through the tricuspid valve during the relaxation phase of the heart cycle—or diastole—the blood enters the right ventricle, the lower right chamber of the heart. Contraction—or systole—of the right ventricle sends blood through the pulmonary valve into the pulmonary artery. This blood goes to the lungs, where it is oxygenated, and returns via the pulmonary vein to the upper left chamber, or left atrium. Contraction of the left atrium—which also occurs during diastole—pushes blood through the mitral valve into the left ventricle, the largest and most powerful chamber. Finally, the left ventricle's powerful final contraction propels blood into the aorta and through the body. A given red blood cell can make this round-trip thousands of times a day, through a network of blood vessels and capillaries that is estimated to be almost one hundred thousand kilometers in length. In a lifetime, the average heart pumps enough blood to easily fill three supertankers.

Harvey would have been touched by the sight of Joseph's heart beating away, its function so obvious when exposed in the bright lights. "It is just as I thought," he might have murmured. Even the cardiac surgeons, who likely saw hearts beating live every day, paused to admire Joseph's heart. For the briefest moment, I could faintly hear the valves within Joseph's heart opening and closing, *lub dub lub dub lub dub*.

"Infusing," called a surgeon and, abruptly, gallons of a refrigerated, clear fluid were injected rapidly into a large vein in Joseph's leg and gallons of his blood drained into a plastic bag from a tube in his chest. The surgeons were replacing Joseph's entire blood supply with a saltwater preservative. *I am watching a boy die*, I thought, feeling a chill as though my own blood were replaced by ice water. *He's already dead, his brain died days ago*, a voice answered. But the chill remained.

Joseph's heart shuddered. The first of the icy preservative entered the chambers. The heart paused for a second to ponder the new fluid within its chambers. Suddenly it recognized the betrayal. Instead of beating in orderly waves, the heart experienced a mutiny; sections began contracting and relaxing randomly. Joseph's heart took on the appearance of a bag of snakes wriggling to get free. This situation is called fibrillation, a state of disorganization caused by confusion of the heart's electrical signaling system. Shortly the heart surrendered completely and lay in Joseph's chest, deflated.

Joseph's body had finally joined his brain in death. His heart stopped when there was no longer any reason to pump, no longer any oxygen to circulate. A heart can't beat, it seemed, without something nourishing to fill it. I thought again about Harvey, who in some sense stripped the heart of its metaphors when he found it was only a pump. Yes, I thought with a sense of loss, looking at the limp muscle that was beating moments ago, it was just a pump.

Using the preservative, the surgeons had placed the heart in a state of suspended animation, stunned but not dead. After another half hour of work, they placed the harvested heart in a foam container for transportation to Pittsburgh.

"Would you like to do the closure?" the chief surgeon asked me. Medical students are often asked to suture incisions after a major surgery was completed. I nodded yes.

"Hurry up," called the surgeon, but I felt a strange sense of obligation to close the wound perfectly, with an under-skin stitching that made the incision almost imperceptible. I don't know why I considered this so important, since Joseph was being cremated anyway. Over the next thirty minutes, I made stitch after painstaking stitch as if Joseph's soul depended on my hiding the empty place where a heart used to be.

Two years later, just before graduating from Johns Hopkins, I was flying to Tokyo on Valentine's Day to work with a team of pediatric cardiologists. At one point my chest twinged as the plane dove. Turbulence, announced a tinny speaker above my head, nothing to worry about. I worried anyway. For a few moments afterward, my heart clanged insistently against my chest. That's the "fight-or-flight" response, I thought distractedly.

In crisis situations, the brain activates specific nerves to telegraph a panic message. A key recipient of the signal is the adrenal gland, a short-fused blob of flesh above the kidneys that responds by spurting adrenaline into the bloodstream, which ultimately gets the heart to pick up the pace. It's all kind of like a fire drill; you go through it many times just to make sure you're prepared for real crises, though these rarely occur.

The heart is a highly disciplined organ, performing its task over and over again. The kidneys produce urine, but also regulate blood pressure, help mineralize bones, and even determine the amount of blood the bone marrow makes. The liver makes cholesterol, detoxifies wastes, and makes salts to break down fats. The pancreas regulates body sugars and makes a bevy of substances to help us digest foods. But the heart more or less pumps blood day in and day out, without engaging in extraneous activities. In a sense, it was fitting that I would study pediatric cardiology in Japan, where medical education is as regimented as the beating of a heart.

The night of my arrival, I met Professor Kazu Koike, the chief of pediatric cardiology at a medical school outside Tokyo. Koike had an infectious grin and welcoming manner. We sipped thimbles of sake, warmed Japanese rice wine, which burned in my chest. After ten minutes, I felt a buzzing in my ears and haziness in my brain. I was tipsy. The beverage had no discernible effect on Koike, who told stories for two hours as I struggled to focus on his blurred outline. At last he left. Before turning in for the night I reflected on the curious intensity with which the Japanese approached both work and leisure. Unlike a heart, Professor Koike seemed not to require periods of diastole, or rest.

In the morning Koike met me in the children's ward of the Saitama Hospital. "Pediatric cardiology," he said, "is based on understanding errors in development of the fetal heart." Koike approached his work seriously and lectured with economy. Around the third week after conception, he explained, a fetal heart develops from the coordinated rotation of a tube of cells. It's an enormously complex series of movements, like those used by carnival performers twisting long balloons into animal shapes. About ninety-nine times out of a hundred, the folding works perfectly, and a normal child's heart results.

A child's heart is the end product of millions of years of evolution. Trees, lacking any mechanical pump, rely on evaporation of water from their leaves to siphon nutrients into their trunks and stems. Fish have a single pump, which sends blood to the gills, from which the blood passes without further pumping to the body. This arrangement has a large performance disadvantage since the gills have high resistance to blood flow. In mammals, the left half of the heart solves this problem by adding a boost to blood returning from the lungs. Koike emphasized that humans have two hearts in one; the right side pumps blood only to the lungs, and the left side takes blood returning from the lungs and pumps it to the rest of the body.

In an unlucky 1 percent of children, the heart isn't formed properly. These children fascinated Koike. As we walked from bed to bed, Koike described the extraordinary diversity of potential heart problems. Anything that can go wrong, sometimes does in fetal development. One child's aorta was hooked to the wrong end of the heart, another baby's heart had a large hole smack in the middle, another failed to pump blood directly into the lungs. And yet these children were alive, adapting. The last child played with blocks, despite the blue color of his face and lips. "You would suffocate if you had the low level of oxygen he has," Professor Koike said to me. "And yet he plays with blocks."

The neurologist Oliver Sacks writes that the joy of doctoring comes not from concentrating on a patient's disorder but on his adaptation to the problem. Children have enormous physiological resilience. They frequently have enormous psychological resilience. Over the years I have grown to love pediatric medicine for this reason: it suggests to me that no problem is insurmountable. There in the cardiac ward, I was seeing a child do the impossible, living with an oxygen concentration previously unimaginable to me. And he was playing with blocks.

A small Japanese infant slept under blue sheets as I readied the large needle. Outfitted like a latter-day samurai warrior, I was already sweating under the lead coat that weighed on me like a suit of armor. Most of the perspiration, though, had nothing to do with my apparel. I was just nervous since I had never done this before. I fingered the catheter and waited for the go-ahead from Koike. We were about to perform heart surgery without touching the heart.

The boy, Domo Korematsu, was three months old and had been noted by his pediatrician one month previously to have an unusual rushing sound in his heart. Domo's heart, like a normal child's, made the typical *lub-dub* sound anyone could appreciate with a stethoscope. But there was also something that didn't belong, an extra rush between the *lub* and the *dub*, like someone blowing air through the chest.

That sound is called a murmur. Imagine standing by a small stream of water flowing through a straight, flat bed of sand. The stream likely flows quietly. Now imagine the stream flowing in a curved path, over pebbles and branches. Here, the stream makes babbling noises because the flow is more turbulent. Blood traveling through the heart behaves the same way. A heart murmur means the blood isn't flowing in an organized manner. In the vast majority of children, turbulent flow is a normal sound associated with a growing, healthy heart. The sounds usually disappear sometime after infancy.

To decide which children's murmurs indicate a heart defect, one has to listen for other clues. To the trained ear a heartbeat is a diagnostic fugue. A small trill, an extra reverberation, or a miniscule click provides important supporting information about possible structural problems with the heart. The heart is a very public organ. Almost every event that occurs—blood entering a chamber, a heart valve opening or closing, or an extra blood vessel where it shouldn't be—leaves acoustic evidence that can be collected with a stethoscope.

These sounds are difficult to describe, and many medical textbooks resort to curious analogies. For example, in his classic treatise *The Art and Science of Bedside Diagnosis*, Joseph Sapira offers the following advice to the budding clinician:

> The murmur of aortic stenosis [a common valve problem] has been likened to the sound of a steam engine chugging up a hill. For prairie dwellers and young persons who have never heard a steam engine on an upgrade, the grunt made by older persons of Mediterranean stock as they settle their arthritic joints into a chair is a passable substitute.

Clearly, direct experience rather than textbook learning is needed to learn the interpretation of heart sounds, and Professor Koike was a virtuoso. He had a theory about Domo's heart. In addition to the murmur, Koike explained, the *dub* of Domo's heart lacked a particular reverberation. Koike thought that Domo had a blockage on the right side of his heart. Koike's prediction was confirmed by an echocardiogram, a type of sonogram of the heart that indeed showed such a problem. (Helen Taussig, the pioneer of pediatric cardiology, had even more impressive diagnostic powers, since she had to make her diagnoses in the 1940s without echocardiograms. Though she became almost completely deaf, she compensated by using her fingers to *feel* the sounds.)

Domo had a traffic jam in his heart. It was as if a six-lane freeway tapered to a single lane. Blood couldn't get out of Domo's heart and into his lungs fast enough due to a condition called critical pulmonary stenosis. Relieving the pressure was an emergency.

"Darshak-*san*," said Professor Koike, interrupting my thoughts, "it is time to begin."

"Yes, Koike-*sensei*." I had adopted some of the formalisms of Japanese names.

We surveyed the area. A large computer monitor at eye level displayed Domo's blood pressure, heart rate, temperature, blood oxygen level, and a continuous stream of Domo's electrocardiogram (the electrical tracing that "flatlines" with alarming regularity on television dramas). These vital signs were comforting. The numbers guarded Domo; if any problem occurred, the monitor would flash red. All of the vitals were currently displayed in a cool blue.

Koike grasped my right hand, which held the large needle, and gradually guided it into the flesh to the right of Domo's groin. Ever so slowly, he urged my hand to push the needle in, millimeter by millimeter. I remembered the first time I had taken blood, in my second year of medical school. We students had to practice on each other. With somewhat nervous hands, I had tied on a tourniquet and swabbed a large vein that materialized in the crook of my partner Jessica's arm. Holding the skin taut over the vein, I inserted a small needle through the skin and Jessica flinched briefly. No blood returned. I advanced the needle without success. Jessica's face tightened and she stared into my eyes, saying nothing. I pulled the needle back and still there was no blood. A small bead of perspiration appeared on Jessica's forehead and her fist clenched. My hand began to tremor. I felt my heart beating in my ears. I advanced the needle again, and suddenly—miraculously!—a flash of red appeared in the syringe. Jessica's hand unclenched.

As Koike guided my hand, I waited for the flash of blood. We continued to advance the large needle. Still, there was no blood. The needle was slightly redirected to the right, and advanced again. No blood. A whistle issued from the vital sign monitor, and the heart rate appeared in red instead of cool blue.

"He's in pain. Stop for a moment," said the anesthesiologist, Taketazu, calmly. Domo was lying sedated on his back, with his arms, feet, and head taped to the table to prevent any accidental movement. He didn't move or seem to wake up when we inserted the needle.

Despite the child's lack of external signs, Taketazu knew that Domo was in pain. In this sense, the work of anesthesiologists is profoundly humane. They must anticipate pain in all forms, especially in those who cannot express pain. Domo was calling out to Taketazu in the only way he could, by speeding up his heart. In operating rooms, some patients show pain only by dilating their eyes or increasing their blood pressure. Anesthesiologists like Taketazu, bringers of comfort, stand watch over those who cannot speak for themselves. Taketazu gave Domo an extra dose of fentanyl, a narcotic similar to heroin, and midazolam, a drug related to Valium. "*Hai*, he is fine," he concluded as the whistling stopped, and the vital signs returned to a reassuring hue.

Koike grasped my hand, and we began again. As we tilted the needle back and advanced, blood shot into the syringe in powerful spurts. "Quickly, thread the wire," Koike said, without a hint of concern. The needle had punctured the femoral artery, which is under high pressure and can bleed enormous quantities quickly. Arteries are gushers.

Like a seamstress, I took the six-inch-long metal wire from Koike and threaded it through the needle in Domo's artery. Gingerly, I extracted the needle, leaving the wire in place. Blood leaked around the wire, and dripped down Domo's side. The wire now served as a guide, which led directly into the artery. Over the wire, I then slipped a hollow plastic catheter, which was thicker than the original needle. I squeezed it into Domo's artery, then pulled out the guide wire, which was no longer needed. I capped the end of the large access catheter with a rubber stopper, and injected sterile salt water with a needle through the stopper. The fluid passed easily into Domo's artery.

We had created an artificial portal into the circulation that led to Domo's heart. Using the same technique, I began again, and this time successfully placed a large catheter just to the side of the arterial catheter. This one went into the femoral vein. Koike looked pleased. "We have achieved access," he said.

What we were performing had first been done in 1929 by an enterprising German physician—and budding crackpot—named

Werner Forssmann. Correctly surmising that a tube inserted into a vein in the arm could get to the heart, Forssmann inserted a long urinary catheter deep into a vein in his own arm, until he thought it reached its destination. (A nurse had tried to stop him from performing this reckless experiment on himself, but he subdued her and tied her to an operating table.) He then walked a flight of stairs to a radiology machine and took an X ray of himself showing that the end of the catheter really had reached his heart. In this bizarre manner, Forssmann performed the world's first cardiac catheterization, for which he later received the Nobel Prize. Cardiac catheterization was important because previously no one could see the heart well, even with X rays. With Forssmann's technique, various dyes were injected directly into the heart, and X rays could then outline structures such as coronary arteries, valves, and heart chambers. Seeing the heart was the first step to understanding heart problems.

Domo's vitals still appeared in cool blue. Koike passed a thin, two-foot-long catheter to me, which I inserted into the femoral vein access catheter, and gradually advanced. With my foot, I pressed a gas pedal–type switch that activated the X-ray machine that took frequent images of Domo's body. These were displayed sequentially on a television monitor like a movie. There were Domo's ribs, sprouting from his spinal column. A pulsating blob in the center of the cage was his heart. Lower down, shadows marked areas where the liver, stomach, and intestines were. On the lower left of the screen, a small white snake inched up, passing the intestines and liver, working its way toward the heart. That was my catheter.

Briefly, the entire image jerked on the monitor. Alarmed, I looked at Koike, who smiled and explained, "Domo just hiccupped, don't worry." I continued to push the catheter, encouraged by Koike. Slowly, I entered Domo's right atrium, the same area of the heart Forssmann had entered almost seventy years earlier. On the monitor, the tip of the catheter moved back and forth, whipped around by the turbulence of Domo's heart. Holding the other end of the catheter, I felt as if I was flying a kite. Instead of wind currents, though, blood currents created the tugging sensations in my line.

"Infusing," said Koike, as he injected a clear dye into the catheter I was holding. Though clear, the liquid contained a chemical that absorbs X rays almost as well as lead. Immediately on the monitor, Domo's heart lit like a firefly as the dye spurted into the right atrium. We saw the path that blood took: the dye outlined the right atrium, where all the body's blood returns to the heart. The dye quickly passed a small tunnel, the tricuspid valve, and entered the spade-shaped right ventricle, just below the atrium. From there, a powerful squeeze propelled the dye into the pulmonary arteries, which sent the blood to the lungs to pick up its cargo of oxygen. It all took less than a second.

"There!" shouted Koike. "Did you see it?"

I didn't. Since the monitor recorded the X-ray images on video, Koike rewound and replayed the sequence. In slow motion, the dye entered the right atrium, passed the valve, and pooled in the ventricle. The ventricle contracted and, instantly, I saw what Koike noticed. The dye leaving the heart outlined an unusual bow-tie shape. Instead of passing through a large open valve, the dye was forced through a constricted exit. The holdup was at the pulmonary valve, which hadn't developed normally. The murmur of Domo's heart was the sound of blood being forced through this malformed valve. It was a bad pipe that needed fixing. Cardiology is a lot like plumbing, and the disciplines share many principles. One would prefer fixing blockages with a noninvasive method like Liquid Drano, rather than tearing down walls and replacing pipes. Similarly, cardiac catheterization is much preferred to open heart surgery.

Koike motioned for me to remove the catheter, and handed another two-foot catheter over to me. This was known as the "balloon." When fluid was injected into one end of the catheter, it entered a balloon at the opposite tip that inflated to the size of a breakfast sausage. The idea was to thread the catheter, with the balloon deflated, into the narrow valve in the heart. Then, we'd quickly inflate the balloon, opening up the narrowing to allow blood to flow freely. It would be a cure.

Ah, a cure—the word sounds so sweet. Physicians lust after cures almost as much as patients. Cures are like proofs of Euclidean theorems: elegant solutions for solvable problems. A cure offers closure, a happy end to an often sad story. Domo was about to get such closure from me. I advanced the balloon into Domo's femoral vein. On the monitor, the tip advanced past the intestines, liver, and stomach, to the right atrium, through the tricuspid valve, into the ventricle, and finally just through the diseased pulmonary valve.

"Inflate the balloon," intoned Koike. Hands shaking, I pushed down on the plunger of the syringe at the catheter end. On the monitor, a small sausage appeared in Domo's heart. Koike waited, counting to himself. "Release the balloon," he requested, and I pulled back the plunger. The sausage disappeared. Koike reached past my hands and pulled the balloon out of Domo's body. After making some measurements to ensure the valve had been repaired, he removed the access catheters as well.

The procedure was over, a success. Though initially excited, I felt somewhat let down. The cure had taken only five seconds to produce. It was minor magic. Surely there were more heroic ways to save children's lives, more serious doctoring to be done.

However, an insatiable hunger for cures is a curse. Take the case of William Halsted. Perhaps no other surgeon had such an illustrious career. The first surgeon-in-chief at Johns Hopkins Hospital, Halsted pioneered thyroid removal and the radical mastectomy, among numerous other procedures. At the height of his career, Halsted graduated 166 chief surgical residents who populated major surgical centers across the country. Medical historian Sherwin Nuland calls him "the greatest surgical scholar our country has ever produced."

But Halsted had a secret. It is unclear if he ever connected emotionally with other people, including his wife. Despite his enviable prowess, Halsted appeared to lack joy. For decades, he turned to cocaine and morphine despite the warnings of his friend, the renowned physician William Welch. Perhaps Halsted was unable to touch his patients' souls, though he opened their chests with his scalpel. I suspect that he could define himself only as a warrior fighting an unseen power of disease, with the patient's body as a battlefield.

In the epic Hindu poem *Mahabharata*, the god Krishna tells the warrior Arjuna that all living things complete repeated cycles of birth and death, until bad karma is exorcised from the soul. In a metaphorically similar manner, patients see caregivers at many visits, dealing with sickness in its many incarnations. The work of a healer is never complete. Perhaps Halsted never realized that healing is a journey and not a destination. Medicine is a poor profession for those who require clear end points or closure in their work.

Koike smiled at me as we left the procedure room, clearly satisfied with the outcome of the procedure. The procedure wasn't really a complete cure, he said. Domo would still require frequent tests to ensure that the problem didn't come back. "It's just the beginning," Koike said.

We stopped in Koike's office to pick up a plastic model of a heart. Then we turned and walked to the waiting room to see Domo's family, where we used the model to explain what we had done to Domo's heart.

Like a heart, life requires a certain cadence, with alternating periods of systole and diastole. Cardiac tissue is a curious mixture of nerve and muscle fibers, a fusion of electrical anticipation and muscular release. Cardiac nerves are molecular clocks that keep time by shuffling charged particles, or ions, of calcium, potassium, and sodium across their cell membranes. Ion by ion, an electric charge builds up, as millions and millions of ions gather. Then, suddenly, one more ion is simply too many, and a point of no return is reached. The pressure is too great. The nerve suddenly lets the ions all crash back in, causing an electrical current to fire into the heart's muscle. Systole has begun, and the heart contracts.

Sometimes I feel like one of these fibers. Medical training, full of classroom hours, wrenching overnight shifts, and the stench of disease, instills in one a longing for liberation. Generally, I keep these impulses at bay, but like the ions around the heart nerves the urges periodically accumulate and become so powerful that I feel ready to burst. I need release.

Systole can take many forms in these situations, some of which are not constructive. Stress drives many doctors in training to substance abuse; a published study of my own residency program found that several trainees had behaviors suggesting alcoholism. Several years ago one Boston Children's resident secretly developed an addiction to narcotics, stealing and self-administering them when on call. One night, he failed to respond to repeated beeper calls. A colleague found him unresponsive in a call room. Tragically, he had died of a self-administered overdose. Resident release could also take other forms. Samuel Shem, in his not-so-fictional bestseller *The House of God* (it is an open secret that it deals with his training at Beth Israel Hospital, across the street from Children's), describes in detail the sexual abandon of residents, seeking brief moments of systole.

In certain open infected wounds, a bacterium called *Clostridium tentani* can grow. This organism produces a unique toxin that causes muscle cells to fire uncontrollably, in continuous systole. These contractions are called tetanic, and the name of this condition is tetanus. The common term "lockjaw" refers to the uncontrolled clamping of the masseter, or jaw muscle. The same situation occurs in several muscles in the body, and the condition can be lethal (about sixty Americans per year die of tetanus). Diastole is critical to survival. Muscles need rest between periods of intensity.

So do people. Many pediatricians, for example, understand that no matter how good you are, you get only two tries to obtain blood from a child before having another one try. After two times, especially on a screaming, restrained child, even the best doctor loses his edge; a fresh pair of hands is needed.

Diastole is sometimes needed on a large scale, too. After my work in Japan, I was feeling somewhat burned out. Medical school was finally over and I needed some way of marking the end of one phase and the beginning of the next. For four months before beginning residency, I satisfied my wanderlust by traveling through Southeast Asia and India, rarely thinking medical or molecular thoughts. I got engaged to my longtime girlfriend, Elizabeth. And I spent long evenings talking with my father, who told meandering stories about his childhood.

The summer after studying in Japan, I began my residency at Children's Hospital, Boston. On my first day as a real doctor, my future depended on memorizing a jingle, which went "Shock, shock, shock! Everybody shock! Little shock! Big shock! Shock, shock, shock!" The song was pretty catchy, and more important, it might have saved fourteen-year-old Antonio Gaudi's life two months later. But I'm getting ahead of myself.

Along with thirty other fledgling doctors, I started a few days of orientation before beginning work at Children's Hospital, the pediatric teaching hospital of Harvard Medical School. We congregated in a large conference room with small babies located at every table. The babies didn't move or make any noise and we shortly realized they were made of plastic. "Welcome to Pediatric Advanced Life Support, or PALS," announced a stocky blond man from the front of the room. PALS is the first thing all residents have to learn and last thing they are permitted to forget.

PALS is a souped-up version of the kind of cardiopulmonary resuscitation taught to the lay public. The principles are quite simple: life-threatening illnesses, including infections, heart defects, and severe seizures, can kill a child by making it impossible to get oxygen into the vital organs. In PALS, we learn how to use a person's built-in ventilation system—the heart and lungs—to restore oxygen to deprived areas of the body. Like the snake oil sold by charlatans to cure whatever-ails-you, PALS is crude medicine because we use the identical techniques on all comers, regardless of the illness. But there is one important difference between snake oil and what we were about to learn: PALS actually works.

Though modern resuscitation was invented only about forty years ago, attempts at saving patients with no heartbeat had begun over a century earlier. In 1887, an enterprising surgeon named Langenbuch noted that his patient's heart had stopped beating under chloroform anesthesia. At the prophetically named Lazarus Hospital, Langenbuch responded by cutting open his patient's chest and squeezing the heart with his bare hands. His patient died, but not before Langenbuch noted that some of the patient's face had recovered its color. That same year, the German physician Kraske performed the world's first successful pediatric resuscitation, saving a five-year-old boy whose airway had closed from an attack of croup. Instead of cutting open the child's chest, Kraske used a new method of external cardiac compression proposed by the Englishman John Hill. Despite Kraske's success, physicians worldwide continued to perform the open chest technique, which invariably created a futile bloodbath.

In the early twentieth century, electric companies funded research on resuscitation of people whose hearts had stopped from electrocution. This work culminated in the electric defibrillator, a shocking device used to jump-start stunned hearts. Later, medications like epinephrine and others were added to the protocol for resuscitation. In 1960, a landmark study by Kouwenhoven demonstrated that closed chest compression, mouth-to-mouth breathing, and electrical defibrillation could deliver a 70 percent "permanent survival" rate. Kouwenhoven felt his method was so simple and so revolutionary that he wrote, "Anyone, anywhere, can now initiate cardiac resuscitative procedures. All that is needed are two hands." His study is generally regarded as the first of the modern era of resuscitation. Although other methods of chest compression have been proposed (one technique, active compression-decompression CPR, was developed after a man successfully resuscitated a family member with a household toilet plunger), none has replaced the chest massage method of Kouwenhoven.

Over the next six hours of the course, Dr. Casey Wygand reviewed the basic principles and practice of PALS. In small groups, the residents rotated from station to station. At the first table, I placed a breathing tube into the windpipe of a disembodied plastic baby head. At the next, I jammed a thick metal needle into a simulated infant leg bone. We then broke to lunch on sandwiches served in picnic-style paper boxes, and I somewhat absentmindedly dissected my sandwich. Returning to the stations, I practiced chest massage on an infant and toddler doll.

At the final booth, Dr. Wygand explained the management of various types of cardiac arrest. In any arrest situation, cardiac monitor leads should be attached to a child's chest. Dr. Wygand held up copies of various squiggly tracings of heart rhythms, printed from actual cardiac arrests. "This one is asystole," he said, showing a tracing of a flat line. "You already know what to do for that one, initiate chest massage and give epinephrine to get the heart going." We had discussed this one earlier. Then, he held up strips of wild seismic patterns, with lines that oscillated without any pattern. "That's ventricular fibrillation," he said. I pictured the harvest of Joseph's heart I saw years earlier, where it briefly writhed like a bag of snakes. The wild tracing fit the condition well. "You fix that condition, you restore normal rhythm"—here Dr. Wygand held up an orderly strip of a normal heart beating—"and I promise you, you'll feel a rush you could never imagine. You'll feel invincible." He demonstrated the technique: First, administer electric defibrillation at two joules per kilogram of body weight, then two further shocks with twice the energy. If that fails, give epinephrine, and defibrillate again. If that fails, give one milligram per kilogram body weight of lidocaine, and shock again. And if that doesn't work, try again with five milligrams per kilogram of a drug called bretylium, and "buzz," or shock, again. Then shock again three times. My head was swimming. How could a person ever remember that, especially in a high stress situation?

"It's easy to recall," said Dr. Wygand. "It's like a cheer: Shock, shock, shock! Everybody shock! Little shock! Big shock! Shock, shock, shock!" It was a mnemonic. The *E* from "Everybody" is for epinephrine, the *L* from "Little" is for lidocaine, and the *B* from "Big" is for bretylium. So much of medical school had been spent memorizing mnemonics; there was simply no other way to remember long lists. There was even an entire book of medical mnemonics that some students used to help study. (To this day, I remember the twelve cranial nerves with the phrase "On old Olympus tilted top, a Finn and German vault a hop.") I mentally added Dr. Wygand's jingle to my collection.

After a few more lectures, the course was over and we were certified to practice PALS. "Go out there," Dr. Wygand concluded by way of a valedictory, "and save some lives."

A nurse sprinted by me to a red cart down the hall. "It's Antonio!" she cried. As residents, we rotated to various areas of the hospital each month and this was my turn on the cardiology floor. At the nursing station I quickly looked to the monitors that displayed the heart rhythms of all the patients. Ominously, Antonio's was displayed in red.

Antonio Gaudi was born with a broken heart. His condition was called transposition of the great arteries, or TGA. Because of confused connections, his heart pumped oxygen-containing blood from the lungs right back to the lungs instead of to the body. A complex operation shortly after his birth, the Mustard procedure, had restored normal connections. But the process had damaged some of the delicate neural wiring of Antonio's heart, and he had required a pacemaker to keep his heart beating in regular rhythms. Over the past few years, his heart's electrical connections had become progressively more dysfunctional.

As if it were recording a seismic event, Antonio's monitor displayed a wildly undulating pattern. With a jolt, I recognized it as ventricular fibrillation. My legs broke into a run that carried me to Antonio's room. He lay in his bed with a glazed expression. I reached for his wrist to feel his pulse, as the nurses readied a medication tray and summoned the attending cardiologist.

Briefly, Antonio's eyes met mine. He grasped my hand and put it to his heart, and he looked as if he were about to speak. Suddenly, he lurched back in his bed as if kicked in the chest by a mule, and simultaneously I felt a crackling burst through the hand placed on his chest. I had just been shocked!

Antonio's pacemaker sensed when his heart was in an unstable rhythm, as it was now. It automatically administered a shock directly into his heart (and now, mine). In a sense, my own heart was now synchronized with Antonio's; we were jump-started at the same moment, joined for a few moments in time. Antonio, now conscious, began yelping in fear. He knew what that shock meant.

Shock, shock, shock! Everybody shock! I thought. Antonio needed epinephrine. "Can I please have epinephrine, five cc's of one in ten thousand?" I asked a nurse. Instantly, a syringe appeared in my hand. I swabbed Antonio's intravenous line with an alcohol wipe and injected the fluid, almost stabbing myself in the finger since my hands were shaking. Clara and Ann, the floor nurses, had already begun wheeling Antonio's bed out of the room as I ran alongside. We had to get him to the cardiac intensive care unit. They soothed Antonio with murmurs of encouragement as we hurtled down the hall. Antonio again appeared to be kicked in the chest, then again. Little shock, I thought. "Can I please have lidocaine, fifty milligrams?" I asked. My hands again slammed the syringe into the intravenous line. Another invisible mule kicked Antonio, and he began to cry.

The door to the cardiac intensive care unit opened, and two attending cardiologists and four nurses took the bed and Antonio from us. "Thanks," said John Moller, the senior cardiologist. "We'll take it from here." I briefly reviewed what happened and walked back to the ward alone. The monitors of the remaining patients were all cool blue. I could feel my heart beating, no longer in synchrony with Antonio's. That was the nature of resuscitations, I guess. You had to let go. Gradually the excitement of the moment diffuses and is replaced by a longing for closure. How was Antonio's story going to end?

I was late. Usually I walked to the hospital since I lived only two miles away. Today, Elizabeth was driving me on her way to work, since I had slept through my alarm. Impatiently, we waited at the intersection of Longwood and Brookline Avenues, just before the hospital. Through a sleepy haze I heard Cory Flintoff announce the morning news on National Public Radio.

Someone dropped from the sky right in front of us.

"Oh my God!" yelled Elizabeth. A teenage girl had been struck by a speeding car, thrown fifteen feet high, and deposited in front of our car. I jumped out of the car, and went to her. She lay on her side, unconscious, with her legs at an odd angle. My mind seemed to have jammed; outside the hospital, I wasn't used to thinking medically. I had no equipment save a pediatric stethoscope. Out of the corner of my eye, I saw Elizabeth talking rapidly into a cell phone. The sedan that struck the girl had stopped. The windshield was smashed and the hood sported a large dent, as if the car had just struck a deer.

Airway, Breathing, Circulation, offered my brain. I listened to the girl's lungs with the stethoscope and heard air move, a beautiful sound. Her heart was beating strongly. I didn't see an obvious head injury. *First, do no harm,* I thought. All I could do was hold her neck immobile and prevent a potential neck fracture from damaging her spinal cord. At the busy intersection, cars waited and their drivers watched a lone physician hold a critically ill girl's head, and do nothing else. Some honked, perhaps hoping the noise would defibrillate her into health. A small ring of bystanders gathered.

The sun shone brightly, gradually clearing the morning mist. I waited. I lay on my belly, holding my arms straight in front of me to grasp the girl's shoulders. Her head was braced securely between my elbows. I looked down directly on her face, so close that her hair periodically grazed my cheek when the wind blew. Though unconscious, she continued to breathe. I waited.

The ambulance arrived, and crisply dressed paramedics took over. They applied a neck collar, shifted the girl onto a stiff transport board, wheeled her into the vehicle, and drove off. It took less than a minute. I returned to the car, and the National Public Radio announcer was still speaking. "Do you think she's okay?" Elizabeth asked, shaken. I had no idea, I answered, and I'd like to know, too. But I never saw the girl again.

"Why are we doing this?" whispered Amy Redd, as we sprinted to the chronic ward. "What's the point?" Every resident knew the patient we were running toward. Jose Rivera was a three-year-old born with a severe encephalocoele, a birth defect that left only the primitive centers of the brain stem intact. He had no conscious brain. Day after day, he lay motionless in a bed, doing nothing, saying nothing, and almost certainly feeling nothing. In contrast, his heart and lungs were perfectly formed and continued to function, keeping themselves alive. Because a brain is critical in regulating certain salts in the body, Jose periodically had bizarre salt concentrations in his blood. This led to periodic cardiac arrests, which was why Amy and I were running to him now.

Jose was born out of wedlock to a teenage Dominican mother named Maria, who under family pressure married the child's father, Roberto. "Jose is my cross to bear," Maria once said resignedly, "say my mother and Roberto." (A social worker also noted that the disability check Jose furnished monthly was the family's most reliable income.) Jose's mother and father wanted every possible heroic measure taken for their child. He had a feeding tube placed directly into his stomach, a special ventilator tube placed through his neck into his healthy lungs, and an orthopedic wheelchair built so he could be brought places. He had spent over half of his life in the hospital. And we were to resuscitate him always, using any means necessary.

When we arrived at Jose's room, other doctors had already initiated chest massage, secured intravenous access, ventilated with oxygen, and attached monitors. The mood was desultory. Jose's parents were out of town, and the unit clerk tried to call them. As always, though, Jose recovered his heart rate and the monitor showed an orderly wave. He was back. "The kid is indestructible," muttered one resident, looking at the tracing. "He'll never die."

Cardiac arrest patients have a 10 to 20 percent survival rate, and advanced life support is thought to be helpful only if initiated within six to twelve minutes of arrest. (Interestingly, one study showed that on television, cardiac arrest patients have a 75 percent rate of survival.) In pediatrics, resuscitation is even more difficult due to the small size of children's bodies. A study demonstrated that paramedical personnel successfully intubated children only half the time, and secured intravenous access only a third of the time. Jose seemed to defy probability. Amy and I returned to our ward. "Why don't his parents let him go?" she said, frustrated. "Can't they just get some closure in their lives and move on?"

A month later Jose arrested again. As usual, he was revived successfully.

Occasionally I am afforded a measure of closure, a needed helping of diastole. Some time after repairing the empty chest of Joseph Abel, the young man who died of a motorcycle accident, I ran into the chief cardiac surgeon, John Watley, who supervised the case. I asked him what became of Joseph's heart after it went to Pittsburgh.

The surgeon in Pittsburgh was relatively new, Watley said, and had reported the procedure in unusual detail in his follow-up note. The Pittsburgh surgeon explained how he had placed a twenty-two-year-old man with heart failure on a bypass machine, and removed the old heart. He described the many connections he made between Joseph's heart and its new host. Finally, he described how the heart was gradually warmed to normal body temperature, and concluded, "The heart came to life right on cue, as if it were still in the host."

~ 3 ~

Blood

ON THE PATH TO REDEMPTION

My father settled into the dining chair and panted, exhausted by his walk from the living room. His oxygen requirements had increased dramatically over the past few months. Now he always wore a long plastic tube that, like an umbilical cord, connected him to the oxygen compressor upstairs. He smiled wanly at my mother and chewed some of the fried flatbread she had made for breakfast. Suddenly he coughed and a small stream of blood poured from his nose.

"*Loi,*" breathed my mother, reverting to her native language as she did under stress. Several drops fell from my father's nose and splashed into his tea. This was his third nosebleed in a week, caused by the dry mucous membranes of his nose from the oxygen flow. I quickly retrieved a paper towel from the kitchen and held his nose closed. He silently gazed at me and waited for the bleeding to stop. The blood bound us together and underscored an irony: in taking my father, the illness created many opportunities for intimacy.

Clotting is a complex process. Over the next ten minutes the smallest blood cells, the platelets, congregated in my father's nose. They clumped and formed a small plug that blocked further bleeding. The spread of scarlet through the paper towel slowed and my father's eyes calmed.

Blood is composed of three major components: the clotting system (which stopped my father's nosebleed), the red cells, and the white cells. These will be explored in turn in this chapter.

Gabe Small's mother, Lily, managed a cooperative grocery store and was skeptical about many aspects of modern medicine. She insisted on a home birth. The decision didn't surprise Lily's midwife, who had once pleaded with her patient to get another measles vaccination since blood tests showed no antibodies. (This is common since the immune response from childhood shots may wane with time, especially with measles vaccine.) But Lily refused.

When she entered labor, she called her midwife but delivered so quickly that Gabe was already crying when the midwife arrived. The midwife dried the infant, cut the umbilical cord, and placed the naked infant on Lily's belly. Briefly she asked if Lily would consent to the routine shot of vitamin K given to all newborns. No thanks, Lily replied. A few hours after the midwife left, Lily held Gabe and walked around the forest behind her house. Everything had seemed so perfect, she told me later.

Over the next three days, Lily blearily went from sessions of breast-feeding to diaper changing and occasionally stole a few minutes of sleep. Though not entirely sure, she thought Gabe was looking a little pale. Likely nothing, she thought. But on the fourth day she knew something was wrong. Gabe's stools, previously the color and texture of mustard, appeared tarry and sticky. And the child now seemed distinctly ashen. Lily called her pediatrician and obeyed his instructions. She wrapped the baby in his papoose and drove immediately to the emergency room.

Gabe could be bleeding rapidly into his stomach, the pediatrician had said to Lily. When subjected to acid—such as hydrochloric acid from the stomach—blood is split into components that appear black and give the stools a telltale color. Because a healthy newborn possesses less than one cup of blood, the loss of even a few tablespoons could prove disastrous.

Blood inspires awe universally. It is an integral ingredient in many creation myths. The Aztecs believed that humans were created from the blood of the divine serpent Quetzalcoatl, and the Norse believed that the vast oceans were the blood of the mythological giant Ymer. Cultural practices worldwide incorporate the imagery of blood. In some Hindu weddings a groom applies a drop of his blood to his betrothed's forehead as a symbol of his lifelong commitment. To ensure the holiness of their foods, Jews and Muslims have rituals governing the bleeding of slaughtered animals. In many religions, blood can symbolize both life and death. Asclepius, the Greek god of healing and the son of Apollo, bestowed life or took it away using the blood of monstrous Gorgons. Christians view the blood of Christ as the most consecrated of sacraments, the promise of eternal life arising from death. Our language today demonstrates continued fascination with blood; blood oaths are the most sacred trusts, blood money the most ill-gotten gains, and blood brothers the most inseparable of companions.

This historical reverence for blood has a solid physiological foundation. One cup of blood distributes a cup's volume of oxygen gas to the body. In a sense, the lungs and heart exist only to ventilate and pump blood. Serious bleeding is every bit as deadly as cardiac arrest or suffocation. Luckily, blood has a way of protecting itself. It can clot.

To grasp Gabe's problem, it is important to understand the components of blood. A complex substance, blood can readily be separated into three distinct layers by a centrifuge. Red blood cells settle to the bottom like sand in a bucket of water. This percentage—about one-third to one-half of the total blood volume—is known as a hematocrit. Just above this crimson layer is a miniscule halo containing the white blood cells, or immune defenders of the body. Finally the top layer, or plasma, is an ale-colored liquid that contains the platelets and dissolved proteins, called factors, that make clots. Until a signal for clotting is received, these platelets and factors remain in a dormant state.

The origins of clotting were poorly understood until about a century ago. In an 1882 article in the British medical journal *Lancet*, Bizzozero suggested that platelets were responsible for initiating blood clots. In 1926, scientists at the University of Montreal confirmed his findings and popularized the idea that platelets were the circulating protectors of the blood. Injured blood vessels release a distress signal that attracts platelets. In response, the platelets gather and clump together, creating a gummy mesh that prevents further blood loss. It's reminiscent of flooding zones in small towns where hardy volunteers quickly arrive to lay down walls of sandbags as temporary barriers. But though somewhat effective, these patches are weak and offer no permanent protection.

Researchers soon found how this rudimentary dam is strengthened. When platelets aggregate, an extraordinary chain reaction occurs. Within seconds, tens then hundreds then millions and then trillions of proteins are activated near the initial bleed. These activated factors deposit a material called fibrin around the platelets. If platelets are the bricks of a clot, fibrin is the mortar.

Back at the emergency room, the triage nurse was alarmed by

Gabe's appearance and immediately had him brought back to see me, the resident on call. I glanced at the vital signs recorded by the triage nurse and saw that his heart was racing. When one doesn't have enough blood to circulate, the heart compensates by pumping faster. Gabe also appeared pale and tired. Usually newborns cry in protest when examined, but Gabe didn't seem to care. When his fingernails were depressed briefly and let go, it took almost six seconds for the color to return. This delayed "capillary refill" meant that his bloodstream was depleted. I inserted a gloved finger in Gabe's rectum and rubbed the tarry stool onto a special card. A drop of reagent caused the stool to turn a brilliant blue: a positive test for remnants of blood. There was no doubt that Gabe was losing a lot of blood.

Anticipating a blood transfusion, I inserted one IV into the crook of his right arm, then another in his left. From the IVs I extracted some blood to check the child's blood type, hematocrit, and clotting status. A "babygram," an X ray of Gabe's entire torso, was normal. I discussed Gabe with the supervising physician and we agreed that the infant urgently needed a blood transfusion.

I spoke with Lily to review Gabe's medical history. He was a full-term infant with no prenatal problems. No family members had ever experienced bleeding problems, including the men on Lily's side. This was important to know since hemophilia A or clotting factor VIII deficiency—the same bleeding disease that affected the doomed royal family of Russia—is hereditary. (Familial clotting disorders have been recognized for millennia; for example, one Talmudic reference to infant blood loss reads, "If two children of the same mother or one child each of two sisters died as a result of circumcision, circumcision of the third child must be omitted.") I asked if Gabe had gotten his vitamin K shot. With a somewhat perplexed look, Lily replied that she had refused it.

The lab called. Gabe had a normal number of platelets but his hematocrit was only 15 percent, about a third of normal. Additionally, his blood took almost three times the normal duration to form a fibrin clot. I dialed the blood bank and asked them to prepare a unit for transfusion. I explained to Lily the need for transfusion. Immediately, she asked to donate her own blood for Gabe.

In doing so, she volunteered to perform a service similar to Adrian Lambert's in 1908. Lambert's wife had delivered a baby girl, but the girl's nose and mouth had continuously oozed blood (she likely had the same deficiency as Gabe). Lambert secured the services of a French surgeon named Alexis Carrel who had recently moved to New York City. Lambert begged him to help and Carrel consented. In Lambert's apartment using no anesthesia, Carrel made an incision in Lambert's wrist and located the radial artery. He then exposed a vein behind the newborn girl's knee. Using a revolutionary surgical technique, Carrel connected the father's and child's circulations so that the father's blood pumped directly into his daughter's vein. The child recovered her color in a few minutes and the bleeding stopped. In this manner, writes journalist Douglas Starr, "The modern era of transfusion medicine began." The infant named Mary went on to recover and Carrel was awarded a Nobel Prize for his efforts in 1912. In retrospect, we know that Mary was lucky that her father's blood type was compatible; many others who later underwent this procedure had acute reactions to incompatible blood and several died.

For years, this is how transfusions were performed since blood typing wasn't widely used until the late 1920s, and no one knew how to preserve blood for more than a few minutes. The twin discoveries of the ABO blood groups by Karl Landsteiner and citrate preservative by Richard Lewisohn made Carrel's type of surgery unnecessary. Now individuals could receive compatible blood that had been donated earlier by volunteers.

I advised Lily not to donate blood for her son. Before any "directed" donations are permitted, blood is tested for several infections in a process that can take days. As became painfully clear from tainted blood donations that transmitted AIDS in the 1980s, blood can be a reservoir for viruses and other pathogens. Even with screening, the risk of acquiring viral hepatitis, HIV, or another infection is close to one in three thousand. Studies have shown that the risk of infection from related donors is no better than that from screened anonymous ones. It was best to give Gabe prescreened blood from our blood bank, I said, since he needed it right now.

As we were speaking, the blood bank was cross-matching a donor's blood to Gabe's. A technician mixed a drop of Gabe's blood with the donor's and made sure that the blood didn't react. Red blood cells have little molecules with various types of sugar displayed on the outside. People with type A have one kind, people with type B another, and people with type O have neither. Transfused blood must not have any sugars that the recipient lacks, because the recipient will destroy any blood with unknown sugars on it. In Gabe's case, even though both samples were type A, the blood could still be incompatible. Apart from the ABO types, there are almost twenty lesser-known types of sugars, including Rh, Kell, Giblett, E, and so on. Often, blood from different donors just can't get along with the patient's blood. Putting two drops of blood in a little dish is the quickest way to tell if there'll be a problem. Happily, Gabe's blood mixed just fine with the donor's.

The blood bank sent the donor's blood to the emergency room. At the sight of it, Lily became almost as pale as her son. Lily was far removed from the culture of medicine that I inhabited, and the transfusion of blood seemed like the ultimate imposition of my world on hers. I had to give her credit. She signed the consent forms for transfusion without a fuss. "Just make him better. This was all my fault," she confessed.

She had made the connection between my asking about the vitamin K shot and Gabe's bleeding. Just as a parent's love of a newborn can be boundless, so can a parent's guilt at possibly having hurt one's child. "I'm so sorry," Lily said to her son, stroking his head.

Gabe had hemorrhagic disease of the newborn, or HDN, a condition described formally in 1852. Lacking normal clotting ability, Gabe's body couldn't repair minor damage to blood vessels. Such injuries occur constantly in newborns; for example, during delivery the head is squeezed during passage through the birth canal, often causing small brain bleeds of no long-term consequence. In a child with HDN, however, these minor bleeds sometimes extend into catastrophic strokes. As in Gabe's case, a slight tear could occur in the digestive tract during normal feeding, resulting in bleeding into the stomach. There, the blood is dismantled by hydrochloric acid and passed in the stool as tarry material.

In HDN, several types of clotting factors are missing so fibrin cannot be made. The platelets work fine in these children. But without its fibrin mortar, the temporary platelet wall can't dam blood vessel leakage for long. Like Gabe, a child with HDN bleeds for extended periods of time from even minor injuries. In 1929, the German biologist Henrik Dam found that chickens fed a diet lacking certain fats developed a type of HDN. Feeding alfalfa leaves to the chickens abolished this bleeding propensity. Dam soon discovered that the active compound in alfalfa that cured the chickens was 2-methyl-3-phytyl-1,4-napthoquinone or, as he termed it, vitamin K (the letter stood for "Koagulation"). The liver makes clotting factors using a biochemical reaction that requires vitamin K. Without vitamin K, several types of clotting factors can't be made. Dam discovered that HDN was simply vitamin K deficiency.

For a variety of reasons including poor maternal nutrition, about 3 to 5 percent of newborns don't have enough vitamin K and might potentially develop HDN. In the 1940s, pediatricians began giving vitamin K to all newborns, hoping this would reduce the prevalence of HDN. It worked. Since injection rather than oral ingestion of the vitamin led to more rapid response, vitamin K injections became a standard greeting for newborns. The shot is usually given before the baby is handed to the mother for the first time. Today, HDN is almost nonexistent.

To help Gabe, we had to stop the ongoing bleeding by replenishing clotting factors. To do this, we first infused an ounce of donated plasma, which contained the factors Gabe didn't have. The factors immediately allowed him to repair the holes in his blood vessels. Then we gave two milligrams of vitamin K, which would allow him to begin making his own factors within six hours. Finally we treated his anemia by giving red blood cells. Gabe's blood transfusion was three and a half ounces of "packed" or concentrated red cells—a little more than seven tablespoons—that dripped into his IV over two hours. His color improved, becoming more like a blooming rose, then he started crying and fussing, a good sign. He was getting better.

In contrast to this treatment, doctors across the street at Brigham and Women's Hospital were saving lives by doing the opposite thing: interfering with the normal function of vitamin K. That story begins in the 1930s and 1940s, when some enterprising biochemists investigated a curious bleeding disease in cattle. They isolated the causative substance, dicumarol, a toxic agent found in sweet clover eaten by the cows. Soon afterward Karl Link of the University of Wisconsin synthesized a derivative of dicumarol that he christened warfarin, after his sponsor the Wisconsin Alumni Research Foundation. Link correctly surmised that warfarin interferes with the liver's ability to use vitamin K to make clotting factors. Taking warfarin makes it harder for a person's blood to clot. Link went on to make millions of dollars for the university by selling warfarin as a rat poison; a massive dose caused uncontrolled bleeding in rats. In 1945, doctors put the drug to more clinical use by treating heart attack patients with it to prevent clots in coronary arteries. Cardiologists at the Brigham and centers worldwide continue the practice today.

After improving in the emergency room, Gabe was admitted to the pediatric ward for observation. He did well, breast-feeding every two hours and having almost no additional blood in his stools. His illness resolved. The next morning I sat with Lily for a little while and heard about her organic foods market. We talked about tomatoes, her favorite produce. She loved the color of vine-ripened tomatoes and the hint of bitter taste when she bit into them. She described how to plant them, keep away parasites, and how to pick them. "I grow everything naturally. In my garden or my body I don't use anything artificial," she said. I nodded.

This distinction between "natural" and "unnatural" medical treatment has popular appeal. A recent report in the *Journal of the American Medical Association* found that almost 42 percent of Americans use herbal or dietary supplements and visit alternative practitioners, at an expense of $27 billion per year. Like Lily, many bemoan the impersonal care delivered by physicians and subscribe to a belief that herbal remedies or ancient treatments are both more effective and less toxic than modern medicines. Supporters of herbal medicines point to the ancient uses of foxglove plant for heart ailments, chinchona bark for malaria, and coca leaves for altitude sickness. But as Marcia Angell and Jerome Kassirer of the *New England Journal of Medicine* point out, "Therapeutic successes with botanicals came at great human cost." The concept of the controlled clinical trial—where carefully selected patients are given novel medications and then compared to those who either take placebos or undergo the usual therapies—was not accepted until the early 1900s. Before then, dangerous and therapeutically useless practices flourished.

A few years ago, I had a glimpse of this old style of medicine. During a botanical research project in western Kenya, I interviewed ethnic Luo healers about their treatments for *chira*, a common wasting disease. In an area with epidemic rates of AIDS, tuberculosis, and parasitic infections—which all cause wasting—*chira* was a catchall diagnosis employed by village practitioners. Different healers used varying doses of herbs, dissimilar methods of preparation, and an inconsistent nomenclature to identify plants. Given the imprecise diagnoses and conflicting treatments, a systematic evaluation of the herbal remedies was impossible. This didn't stop any of the healers from reporting perfect success. Until the advent of the controlled clinical trial, American medicine had been practiced just like this. (The situation in Kenya was particularly sad because effective treatments for the causes of *chira* were available at a local health center run by the World Health Organization.)

But are the millions of Americans who use "alternative" remedies misguided? This seems unlikely. A reasonable amount of medical literature suggests, for example, that a flower called echinacea effectively treats colds in adults. Is echinacea now an alternative herbal therapy or a modern pharmaceutical? In an effort to frame this debate more constructively, the *Journal of the American Medical Association* editorialized in 1998:

> There is no alternative medicine. There is only scientifically proven, evidence-based medicine supported by scientific data or unproven medicine, for which scientific evidence is lacking. Whether a therapeutic practice is "Eastern" or "Western," is unconventional or mainstream, or involves mind-body techniques or molecular genetics is largely irrelevant except for historical purposes and cultural interest.

Rather then be categorized as "alternative" or "conventional," therapy should be deemed "proven" or "unproven." Educated physicians therefore have no problem when patients use St.-John's-wort for mild depression or acupuncture for certain pain syndromes, but are strongly suspicious of their using "aura fluffing" for cancer or magnets for headaches. Likewise they endorse the proven use of penicillin for strep throat but don't support the unproven practice of restricting sugar intake in children to prevent hyperactivity.

In addition to the imagined incompatibility of "alternative" and "modern" medicine, many physicians resent the metaphysical notion that disease is largely a manifestation of mental or spiritual weakness. Bestselling author Dr. Andrew Weil writes, "Physical manifestations [of disease] are mostly caused by nonmaterial factors, in particular by unnatural restraints placed on the unconscious mind." Clearly, no physician in his or her right mind disagrees that mental well-being is a key component of good health. But it's unlikely that Gabe bled because of "unnatural restraints placed on the unconscious mind." He just didn't have enough vitamin K.

Lily and I had a spirited discussion about these topics. She didn't completely come around to my point of view. But though I doubted she'd ever change her mind about her own use of "natural" herbal products over "unnatural" pharmaceuticals, at least now she was unwilling to stake her child's health on her beliefs.

Lily looked over at her son. "Maybe my next child will get a vitamin K shot," she said.

In the emergency room, Monica Johnson screamed in pain and held her right leg. Sixteen years old, Monica suffered today because of something in her red blood cells that had likely protected her ancestors.

A teenager with considerable tolerance for pain, Monica was continually challenged by her affliction's limitless capacity for agony. As I approached her stretcher, her jaw was clenched and her eyes fixed steadily upward as she struggled to master the madness of her leg. Pain fibers in her leg's nerves fired repeatedly and dumped the chemical acetylcholine onto other nerves, telegraphing a single message through her spinal cord to a place deep in her brain, drenching her consciousness over and over with its brutal impulse: Feel pain, Monica, feel agony. With effort, she turned to me and blinked her eyes as if to say, I'm in control for a moment. She formed one word before the control was lost and she screamed again. The word was, "Morphine."

I rummaged through my lab coat and extracted a deck of code cards, or medical protocols. On sequential index cards, I had printed recipes for various emergency treatments. I flipped past new onset seizures, neonatal fever, croup, and found the card for Monica's problem. Medical practice is a secretly anti-intellectual endeavor; the most successful doctors are those who remember protocols, memorize facts, and build up a lot of experience. The best clinicians are simply the best pattern recognizers. And here I was with my cards, hoping to be one of them, an information dispenser with some compassion.

Monica was certainly right; she needed morphine. She was experiencing a "vaso-occlusive crisis," which meant that the blood in her leg had become sludge. Normal red blood cells are disc-shaped and flow through arteries smoothly. Usually, Monica's cells were also disc-shaped but they maintained the shape tensely, on the edge of collapse like mousetraps. About four times a year it suddenly happened. Monica's red blood cells snapped into sickles and gummed up arteries, usually in her legs. To her, it felt like a tourniquet that couldn't be cut away.

Monica's problem would never have existed if we didn't possess such a wonderfully evolved method of oxygen delivery, red blood cells. Rust on exposed metals and red blood cells get their hue from the same substance, iron, which craves contact with oxygen. Unfortunately, when left together, iron and oxygen couple irreversibly into rust. Therefore, in blood, special antioxidants form a barrier that discourages iron and oxygen from getting too close. After all, oxygen has to be picked up, but also dropped off. The complex of iron and antioxidants is called heme, the body's delivery service for oxygen.

Why, then, don't Monica and the rest of us just have tiny molecules of heme instead of blood cells? Heme binds another gas almost twenty-five thousand times more strongly than oxygen, a poisonous waste made by our cells called carbon monoxide. Any free heme instantly would be monopolized by this poison and unable to carry oxygen. Thus we also evolved a complex protein—a sort of molecular chaperone—to discourage carbon monoxide binding. Four of these bodyguards surround each heme molecule in a tile-shaped pattern, and the collective substance is called hemoglobin.

Unfortunately, hemoglobin, like naked iron, binds oxygen so well that it doesn't let it go even when it reaches the capillaries. So we evolved red blood cells, which possess yet another chemical called 2,3-diphosphoglycerate, or DPG. DPG reduces the attraction of hemoglobin for oxygen by just the right amount. When red blood cells pick up oxygen in the lungs, they are completely saturated. As the cells travel to their final destinations, the bloodstream becomes slightly more acidic. In the presence of DPG, hemoglobin becomes exquisitely responsive to this change and immediately unloads the oxygen cargo. This cascade explains why we have hemoglobin and red blood cells.

I ordered ten milligrams of morphine—enough to flummox a girl twice Monica's size—but it didn't touch her. I gave ten more and an aspirinlike painkiller called ketorolac. We still hadn't exchanged more than one word, which still hung in the air. Morphine. Monica was in no mood to talk, occupied in a battle with pain that could only be fought alone. I found her chart and read through it while waiting for the morphine to infiltrate and soothe Monica's brain.

Monica's hemoglobin was over 99 percent normal, but this wasn't good enough. As in a complex computer program, an error in a single line of code can crash an entire system. When her hemoglobin loses its oxygen under certain conditions, it becomes sticky and gets bound to another hemoglobin nearby. When about ten of them all bunch together in this manner, a chain reaction begins. It's kind of like making rock candy by suspending a piece of string in saturated sugar water; the crystals seem to appear all at once. Monica's red blood cells will suddenly fill with needlelike crystals of hemoglobin. A previously pliable cell becomes a stiff sickle. Circulation becomes impossible, as if one were trying to pump horseshoes through a garden hose. A vaso-occlusive crisis begins and Monica experiences her torture. Only morphine can help her then. We just wait for the diseased cells to fall apart, which can take days.

Five minutes after the second dose, the morphine had taken the edge off Monica's agony and she could talk. Without the pain she was articulate. "Did you ever read *Beloved?*" she asked me. "There's this one scene where a slave is running away, and she spends a night in a shed, but when she wakes up her leg is asleep and it's killing her. This lady comes up to her and massages her leg, and that makes it hurt even more. You know what the lady tells the slave? *Anything coming back to life hurts.* That's what it's like, resurrecting my leg."

James Herrick, a Chicago doctor, discovered Monica's disease in 1904. A twenty-year-old black college student under Herrick's care was admitted to a hospital with fever and a cough. In those days, doctors did most of their own laboratory studies, and Herrick noted a peculiar finding in the student's blood cells under a microscope. Puzzled by what he called "a tendency to the peculiar crescent-shape in the red corpuscles," Herrick became the first to describe a case of sickle cell anemia and published his work six years later.

Herrick extensively described his exam of his patient, and while examining Monica I noticed some of the same findings. A careful physical exam can be a very invasive undertaking, but it can also be healing in its own right. T. Berry Brazelton, a noted specialist in child development, once lectured me on using the physical exam as a means to offer comfort as well as gather information. Thus I wash my hands with hot water first, since children seem to prefer warm hands. All doors are closed and televisions switched off, so quiet prevails. On infants, I learned to massage and gently confine their movements to hear a heartbeat. On older children, I usually begin an exam by carefully observing a child's hands and fingernails.

Monica's hands were rough, and the area under her fingernails was yellow. The tips of her fingers were slightly numb. Previous vaso-occlusive crises in her fingers, which can kill small nerves, likely caused this. I worked my way to her arms, which were fairly thin for a teenager. Typical: sickle cell patients were often thin. From there, I placed the bell of my stethoscope on her breastbone. Monica's breathing was even and deep. I listened for almost a minute, as much to have Monica concentrate on her breathing and retain calmness as for the information it gave me. Her heart slowed somewhat, and I clearly heard a murmur, likely from her blood, which was turbulent due to its paucity of red cells. To my surprise, Monica hummed quietly to herself and the pleasant low buzz complemented her heart's whooshing.

Next, I rubbed my hands together to warm them and placed my right hand just below her rib cage on the right side. As Monica inhaled deeply, I felt the edge of her liver migrate downward. Its smooth contour was reassuring; a hard edge meant liver scarring that occasionally occurred in patients who had frequent sickling events in the organ. I shifted my hands to her left side and gently palpated. I could feel no spleen, which was typical, since sickle cell patients lose their spleens soon after their toddler years. (This was particularly important to know; the spleen is critical in fighting infection from bacteria like *Salmonella* and *Pneumococcus*. Thus all children with sickle cell anemia should take penicillin twice a day to prevent infection.)

I pulled the hospital gown down to cover Monica's belly and turned to her legs. Placing my hand on her left foot, I asked her to point her toe. Then I applied resistance and this time Monica was unable to push me away. This weakness was unusual and meant that Monica had likely suffered a stroke, or crisis in the right side of her brain. This is, unfortunately, also common in sickle cell disease. I desisted from touching her right leg and turned to her face.

Placing my hands on her cheeks, I felt Monica's sinuses with my thumbs, palpated below her eyes, then pressed on her forehead. Taking a lighted eyepiece, I peered into her eyes and looked at the lattice of blood vessels that bloomed behind her irises. The stems of vessels were frayed slightly, another product of untoward sickling. I put the ophthalmoscope away and examined the white of her eyes, which had a golden tint. Sickled cells have a tendency to spontaneously burst, spilling their contents into the bloodstream. The rich scarlet of hemoglobin then degrades to a yellow chemical called bilirubin that dyes the eyes. This condition is called jaundice.

From the moment I began my exam I hadn't broken physical contact with my patient. If one hand was moving the other stayed put on her body. I always do my exams in this way, particularly on patients in pain. To let go before the exam was complete seemed to break a tenuous connection that held us together, and just seemed to keep away the pain. Now finished, I slowly lifted my hands from Monica. Gradually she yielded to morphine, lost in fields of poppies. Monica slept.

In certain parts of West Africa, almost 40 percent of the inhabitants possess the sickle hemoglobin "trait," meaning that their bloodstreams have about half sickle hemoglobin and half normal hemoglobin. These people have one gene for normal hemoglobin from one parent, and one gene for sickle hemoglobin from their other parent. When two persons with the trait mate, they have about a one in four chance of having a child who has two genes for sickle hemoglobin and none for normal hemoglobin, and therefore sickle cell disease. Why, one might ask, is this trait so common?

This problem intrigued biologist Anthony Allison in the 1950s. If the gene for sickle hemoglobin were disadvantageous, natural selection should lead to its elimination over time. There were two possibilities to explain its current prevalence: either the gene was being spontaneously generated—mutating—at a rate one thousand times higher than any other known gene, or sickle hemoglobin conferred some survival advantage. Allison made a map of Africa showing prevalent areas of the sickle cell trait, and noted that these correlated with areas of endemic malaria, especially the deadly form caused by *Plasmodium falciparum*. He hypothesized that sickle cell hemoglobin protected against this disease.

Scientists later discovered how this happens. Cells from people with only the trait and not the full disease—individuals possessing half normal and half sickle hemoglobin—*will* sickle, but only at very low oxygen levels. Malaria is caused by small parasites that infect red blood cells after being introduced into the bloodstream by an infected mosquito's bite. While reproducing in the cells, the parasites consume a lot of oxygen. When the oxygen levels cross the critical threshold, the cell suddenly sickles. It's a mousetrap. The spent cells—and their noxious invaders—are then removed from the body by the spleen. Thus these persons, who have no symptoms of sickle cell disease since they also possess normal hemoglobin, are protected from malaria.

Yet though Africans are three times more likely than American blacks to have sickle cell trait, they are much less likely to have sickle cell disease. One would think that there would be many, many more people with sickle cell disease in Africa since so many prospective parents have the trait. This disparity is due to the early death of Africans with sickle cell disease: half of afflicted children die before age three and fewer than one in ten live past ten years. Nature generally has not intended that these children should live. Poor Monica, I thought, as I watched her sleep. It seemed that some power had designated her expendable. Her suffering was merely collateral damage in our species' struggle to evolve.

So Monica and children like her fight back, with a little help. In America, almost all children with sickle cell disease live well past their teens. Every day Monica takes a tablet of folic acid, a critical vitamin used in the synthesis of hemoglobin. In the summer months, she drinks an eight-ounce glass of water every three hours, since we know that well-hydrated individuals experience sickling less frequently. Because she lacks a spleen, she is immunized against several types of bacteria known to infect such patients, and also takes penicillin tablets twice a day. Four times a year, she meets with a nutritionist who helps improve her diet. Plus, she was about to begin taking a revolutionary medicine called hydroxyurea.

While Monica slept, I wheeled her stretcher from the emergency room to the pediatric ward. The evening nursing shift had come on, and the lights were turned down in the halls. It was remarkably quiet. The admitting nurse joined me and we took Monica to her room. Still asleep, Monica had several monitors attached to her chest, an oxygen tube placed under her nose, and a small box attached to her IV. This box was a patient-controlled analgesia device, or PCA. With a small button placed in her hand, Monica could immediately deliver a dose of morphine to herself if she woke up in pain. Later, I could review the number of times she had dosed herself and quantify the cadence of her pain.

I returned in the morning and Monica looked much better. Wearing wire-rimmed glasses, she looked up from Dante's *Inferno*. "I'm able to walk now," she said. Only a few additional milligrams of morphine were needed overnight. She had jettisoned her hospital gown and today dressed in denim overalls and a painter's cap. "Can I get out of here yet?" she asked. Monica didn't remember much from the night before, because high doses of opiates and other agents such as ketamine can induce a sort of amnesia.

This raises an interesting philosophical dilemma: Is pain only bad if it's remembered? Though a sedated person experiences pain as it occurs, the experience is deleted from memory soon afterward. I've seen children scream while getting broken bones set by the orthopedic surgeon, only to forget the incident several minutes later under the influence of such drugs. One's brain is transported back to the moment before the pain. These wondrous drugs are a kind of time-travel aid.

Like the brain, Monica's blood also needed a time-travel aid. Before Monica was born, she had no sickled cells. A fetus possesses a unique type of hemoglobin that binds oxygen slightly more strongly than normal hemoglobin. The developing child needs to bind oxygen more strongly than its mother or else no oxygen would get from the mother's bloodstream to the fetus's. A few months after the child is born, his or her adult hemoglobin genes take over and fetal hemoglobin production stops. Though Monica had normal fetal hemoglobin, her adult hemoglobin was abnormal sickle hemoglobin. Therefore, she began showing the first signs of sickle cell disease when she was six months old.

The notion that reversing this genetic takeover—turning back the clock on red blood cells—could help patients with sickle cell disease was tested by Samuel Charache at Johns Hopkins Hospital a few years ago. For many years, cancer researchers had found that a chemotherapeutic drug called hydroxyurea has the interesting side effect of increasing fetal hemoglobin production in adults. Charache found that daily administration of hydroxyurea to people with sickle cell disease brought back fetal hemoglobin, and reduced their number of vaso-occlusive crises by an astounding 50 percent. In fact, their study was prematurely stopped since they felt it was unethical to withhold such effective therapy from those receiving only routine care.

Monica went home the next day, discharged from her purgatory with renewed confidence and a vial of white tablets of hydroxyurea. For the last six months of my tenure at that hospital, I didn't see her in the emergency room. Occasionally I ran into the hematologist who saw Monica for monthly checkups. She was doing well, he told me, with no pain crises.

In a sense, Monica was predestined to suffer on the cross of evolution so others of our species could survive. It was therefore fitting that hydroxyurea's renewal of a part of her body—a rebirth of her very lifeblood—gave her salvation from pain.

It wasn't possible to use the showers; the children were simply too dirty. We'd have to use the garden hoses. It was "Down and Dirty Day" at Camp Sunrise where I volunteered as a cabin counselor, and the sixty campers shared the unusual distinction of all having cancer.

The morning had started with Fruit Baseball, and the name explained the activity. One of the staff volunteers owned a wholesale fruit business and donated bushels of outdated tomatoes, apples, nectarines, oranges, and bananas. I pitched. Never, and I mean never, have I enjoyed baseball more. Hit just right with an aluminum bat, the fruits exploded exuberantly and covered the batters with pulp. The children screeched with delight with every hit and my charges shortly resembled fruit salads.

We moved on through a variety of other stations, each messier than the one previous. Egg Toss added another layer to the fruit, which adhered nicely to the subsequent shell of gelatin at Jell-O wrestling. As they dried in the sun, the children began to make crackly sounds as they moved their arms, legs, or faces. Already the children were unrecognizable and the Oatmeal Pool Rescue and Tug of War in the mud pit completed their disguises. Now they resembled shambling mounds, golems of earth.

The problem now was how to clean them off before dinner. Bruce, a research biologist who had dreamed up the whole activity, lined up the children and handed me the hose. "Step right up," Bruce said to the first figure, which must have been only six or seven years old. The child raised his arms and I aimed the hose at him. As the water poured over him a nose emerged, followed by ears, eyes, mouth, and torso. It was little Justin Field, I realized. "Next," called Bruce and another child was born from the dirt mound that approached. That one was Brittany Weams, a ten-year-old girl with leukemia.

As they progressed through the cleansing station, I began to imagine I was sculpting children from earth with the garden hose. Each of them had had a life-threatening condition. Most had leukemia or lymphoma, abnormalities of the blood that were the most common pediatric cancers. A handful had brain tumors, bone growths, or other cancers. Somewhat fancifully, I thought the water was a restorative. From the dirt the water was rescuing children, clean and joyful and healthy. I couldn't keep such magic confined so I doused Bruce and any other staff member who got close. I was dispensing holy water, after all.

The last camper to be freed was Matt Willow, who sported a wicked grin. The day before, his counselors got him a gift that seemed in questionable taste: a vomit basin with alligator decals on it. Matt had an aggressive type of leukemia and was getting a bone marrow transplant in a few days. He was going to need the basin.

Matt was the ringleader among the teenagers I supervised at Camp Sunrise. Though physically smaller than most of the other sixteen- and seventeen-year-olds, Matt had a magnetism that drew them to him. His appeal was based on his wit; he was equally comfortable matching teasing insults at machine-gun speed with his peers and telling sweetly inane riddles to the kindergarteners. In a skit at the talent show, Matt had pretended to be "Simon in the Bathtub," a little boy gurgling jingles as he pretended to take a bath. His songs had children of all ages in stitches. Toward the end, he looked up with a sheepish grin and deadpanned, "Oops! I made some bubbles." This brought down the house.

So Matt was going to get a bone marrow transplant. His story was similar to many of the other children's at camp. One day when he was in elementary school, Matt's mother thought he looked a little pale and brought him to the pediatrician. Because paleness could imply a lack of adequate numbers of red blood cells, the pediatrician checked Matt's complete blood count, or CBC. Matt's hematocrit was only 15 percent, less than a third of normal. That meant that Matt was either losing his blood somewhere or not making enough.

The CBC is a simple test often run in a pediatrician's office and offers a wealth of information. Using a laser beam, the CBC machine counts all the cells in a drop of blood and measures their sizes and their types. That's how Matt's pediatrician knew about the anemia, or lack of red cells. Furthermore, he knew the cells were of normal size and shape, which indicated that Matt didn't have iron deficiency (since the cells weren't shrunken), folic acid deficiency (since the cells weren't inflated), or acute bleeding (since there were no immature, small red cells usually rushed into the circulation during times of blood loss). Matt also had almost no platelets. This was particularly alarming to the pediatrician, especially when he saw that Matt had almost twenty times the usual number of white blood cells. Matt's white blood cells had launched a blitzkrieg on his bone marrow and displaced all the areas manufacturing red cells and platelets. The marrow became a factory for making only one thing: white blood cells. The diagnosis: leukemia.

The cause of leukemia has been studied for decades. Exposures to chemicals like benzene, genetic conditions like Down's syndrome, viruses related to HIV, and radiation can all contribute to higher risks. But the bottom line is that no one knows the cause for sure. At some point in Matt's bone marrow, a single white cell suddenly lost its reproductive restraint. In medical parlance, the cell "transformed." It divided, and the offspring divided again, and so on. The typical leukemia patient has almost *one trillion* of these cells in his body at the time of diagnosis. They keep on dividing, forcing everything in their path away. The marrow fills with cancerous cells. Perhaps that is why cancer is so frightening; its advance seems so inexorable and merciless. (The cancer cells of a woman named Henrietta Lacks, who died in 1951, are so relentless that they survive in laboratories around the world today and still reproduce at a breathtaking pace. These so-called HeLa cells are used to study everything from polio vaccines to cell reproduction. One researcher quipped, "She weighs more now than she did when she was alive.")

Only fifty years ago, leukemia was uniformly fatal and the average afflicted child lived for only two months after diagnosis. Perhaps the best-known leukemia patient at the time was Sadako Sasaki, a two-year-old girl exposed to radiation when her hometown of Hiroshima, Japan, was bombed in 1945. Ten years later she felt dizzy and collapsed at school and was shortly diagnosed with the "A-bomb disease," or leukemia. Sadako's best friend told her of an old Japanese myth that anyone who folded a thousand paper cranes, or *senbazuru*, would be granted a wish. Day after day, Sadako folded cranes but according to legend succumbed to her disease just after she folded her nine hundred and fifty-fifth crane. In memory of her, her schoolmates finished folding her cranes. Some time later, a memorial was erected in Sadako's memory at the Hiroshima Peace Park. When I visited it some years ago, one could barely see the structure for the thousands upon thousands of cranes that children from around the world folded and mailed to Hiroshima.

In a sense, Sadako's classmates' wish for peace and healing was answered. After World War II, some scientists noted that exposure to mustard gas caused bone marrow and lymph node damage. At Yale University in the 1940s, Gilman also noted this effect and thus began using a related compound to treat lymphoma, a type of blood-based cancer where the lymph nodes enlarge. Sidney Farber in Boston induced the first remission in pediatric leukemia soon afterward. Based on these successes, the National Cancer Institute beginning in 1955 oversaw a remarkable program in which over 400,000 substances—everything from plant extracts to ground-up animal parts—were screened for anticancer properties in mice implanted with human tumors. Many promising drugs were identified, and doctors suddenly had access to a vast array of anticancer therapies. Matt certainly lived in a better time to have leukemia than did Sadako.

Over the three months following his diagnosis some of these medications, or chemotherapy, were injected into Matt's bloodstream. Some of these drugs are so toxic that merely touching them with your fingers can induce a burn. Because these chemicals can't enter the brain from the bloodstream, Matt also had chemotherapy directly injected into his nervous system through spinal taps. Like almost 70 percent of children with his type of leukemia, Matt's bone marrow showed no evidence of the cancer after the therapy. Just as Matt's parents remember the horror of his diagnosis, they also remember the day the oncologist announced that Matt had been cleared of the cancerous white cells, or achieved "remission."

Every year Matt returned to see his oncologist, who inserted a large metal needle called a trocar into Matt's hip to extract a small amount of bone marrow. (Matt remembers that the doctor told his parents that the pain felt something like menstrual cramps, an analogy that forever placed him in awe of the fortitude women must possess.) Peering through a microscope, the oncologist looked for any reappearance of the small blue cells of leukemia. Every year for a decade the oncologist pronounced Matt cancer-free. But Matt's luck ended this year. "Your son has relapsed," Matt's parents were told. Several weeks of additional chemotherapy later, Matt's marrow still hadn't responded. "He's failed the therapy," the oncologist reported.

The trillion cells of leukemia had renewed their assault on Matt's bone marrow. In addition to once again displacing the red cells and platelets, normal white cells were also not being made. With normal immune cells absent, bacteria and fungi and viruses had ready access to Matt's body, a fertile land with no defense. These infections are termed opportunistic since they take advantage of a weakened condition. A fungus called mucormycosis, a foul black mold, infected Matt's mouth and his doctors beat it back with an antibiotic called amphotericin B, or, as Matt called it, "ampho-terrible" because of the fevers and nausea it caused. Other infections followed and were narrowly defeated. Matt's doctors fired off a second round of chemotherapy, which beat back the leukemia somewhat but not to remission. It would shortly return.

There was only one way to achieve a cure. One doctor summarized the plan by saying, "When the garden's bad, you have to rip it up and replant." Matt needed a bone marrow transplant. This meant that the doctors needed to destroy every last bit of the marrow—every cell that made the blood and the platelets and the dreaded leukemic cells—and replace it with healthy marrow. The destruction of the leukemia would be performed by the administration of large doses of radiation, the same thing that had given leukemia to Sadako Sasaki. Like the use of nitrogen mustard, this treatment was a curious instance of a sword beat into a ploughshare. In receiving ten Gray units of radiation (an exposure likely five to ten times that Sadako received), Matt's leukemic cells would be blasted apart as they attempted to reproduce. He would be cured of leukemia. But then his problems would intensify.

Before the transplant, Matt came to camp. Maybe Matt wanted to be around a collection of living, breathing miracles, children like Marilyn who had been cured against all odds by a transplant five years earlier. Then there was Mikey, who had undergone two consecutive bone marrow transplants and fought his way back to the ranks of those in remission. And how could one forget Sara or Benjamin or Courtney, who each had equally heroic stories?

Two days before camp ended, I took a picture of Matt that I still look at from time to time. The evening activity was a medieval carnival and several older children dressed in court costumes to entertain the younger children. In the picture, Matt is wearing a jester suit and his face is turned slightly away from the camera. I think he was juggling beanbags, though they were cut off in the picture. His hands are open and stretched out and his eyes are looking upward.

He was caught at a rare moment when he wasn't smiling; instead, his lips are pursed and his face is expressionless. In his jester costume, Matt seems to be longing for something, but also strikes a pose that suggests resignation.

Matt was admitted to the bone marrow transplant unit soon after camp. Because the procedure is so complicated, the transplant runs according to a specific protocol. Each day of the transplant is numbered, as in a space launch. On day T minus five, Matt underwent "conditioning," where the radiation therapy was delivered in a small room the size of a telephone booth. At the moment when the radiation is deployed, the patient feels only slight warmth.

Unfortunately, an irradiated person like Matt then becomes a time bomb. Just as it kills leukemic cells, radiation kills all the stem cells that produce red cells, white cells, and platelets. This is a huge problem because the existing blood cells don't live very long. Though some cells like nerves can live for decades, normal blood cells can die soon after birth. For example, the neutrophil, a critical white blood cell that fights bacteria, lives only one day. Though free of cancer, Matt was left as prey in a jungle of bacteria. Matt's immune system would behave something like Superman exposed to kryptonite; enemies defeated effortlessly in the past become insurmountable. Soon after the white cells are gone, the platelets disappear. A bump on the head could prompt a fatal stroke, and attempts at defecation may prompt horrifying bleeding. Finally, the red cells become extinct and Matt's body might slowly suffocate.

Hence Matt required replacement bone marrow, introduced just after his irradiation. This procedure is called a bone marrow "rescue." After an absolution from cancer, Matt's empty bones would take communion with a new spirit, that of his father.

Matt's father donated the marrow for the transplant. Some days before the transplant, a trocar was inserted into his hip and several tablespoons of pulpy marrow were extracted. In a laboratory, this extract was washed and placed in a salt solution in preparation for transplant. The key components of the marrow are called stem cells, since they may branch down many different developmental paths. Given the right molecular fertilizer, a stem cell can give birth to more stem cells, platelets, red cells, white cells, and even certain bone cells. Like refugees marooned on a lush island, these stem cells can settle into Matt's marrow and—if the host is lucky—make a permanent home, or "engraft." A person who has successfully engrafted has a symbiotic relationship with his new marrow. The marrow extracts nutrition and oxygen from the host's body, and in return manufactures all the blood cells the host needs.

The transplant itself appeared anticlimactic. Sometime in the morning of the transplant, a nurse floated into Matt's room with a wallet-sized bag containing pink fluid. She hung the bag on an IV pole, attached about five feet of plastic tubing, and connected the bag to an IV entering Matt. Smiling angelically, she activated the mechanism of the IV and for about one hour the pink liquid dripped into Matt's vein. When the bag was empty, the nurse smiled again and said, "It's in."

He had just received a bone marrow transplant. Like homing pigeons, stem cells deposited in the bloodstream find their way to the bone marrow to roost. Nobody knows how this works. One theory is that the stem cells pursue a trail of molecular markers—like a police dog who locates a suspect by scent—secreted by the bones.

Successful settling of the bone marrow can take weeks. In the meantime, the recipient must be protected against bleeding, infection, and anemia. Matt would have to live in a bubble. This wasn't literally true, as in the case of the "bubble boy" David Vetter, who lived in one from 1972 to his death in 1984. (He suffered from a rare syndrome called severe combined immunodeficiency.) Instead, Matt stayed in a room where all air was filtered the same as in biocontainment facilities. Visitors had to wash their hands with abrasive soaps before entering, and masks and gowns were required. Every day, Matt's skin was washed with a brown antiseptic called chlorhexadine and his body was filled with antibiotics to prevent the slightest enticements to bacterial colonization. He wasn't allowed to eat any food, since food contained potentially harmful bacteria. A sterilized, liquid nutrition was given through his veins. Every day Matt's blood was checked for bacteria. And, of course, he was not permitted to leave the ten-by-ten-foot containment room. While his marrow regenerated, the idea was to keep Matt as distant as possible from his friends, relatives, other visitors, and even from the bacteria on his body. Though such confinement sounds like an additional torture, successful bone marrow transplantation *depends* on the patient's being separate.

On day T plus eight, Missy (another staff member from camp) and I went to visit Matt. We scrubbed and gowned as instructed before entering. Next to his bed I noticed the alligator vomit basin, which had recently been washed. Matt was noticeably paler and thinner. But radiation and cancer still hadn't dulled his adolescent wit; when a nurse entered the room and asked if he was having any trouble urinating, he answered, "Yeah, my doctor told me not to lift any heavy objects." Used to his antics, the nurse smiled and left.

Toward the end of the visit Matt said to Missy and me, "I need you to do something important for me." Seated at the foot of his bed, we looked up to him for our task. For the hospital room, he wanted a very specific poster of "Kermit Hilfiger," a spoof in which Kermit the Frog models some clothing from designer Tommy Hilfiger. Matt didn't explain why and we didn't ask. We would of course oblige him.

Missy and I picked up Matt's best friend from camp, Paul, and we drove from store to store in search of the poster. It was a tough assignment. Every store clerk asked why we needed the Kermit poster; it was a rare request. We'd tell Matt's story and it always affected them. Like apostles we must have gone to fifteen stores, telling Matt's story to anyone who listened. It was just like him, we laughed, to send us on a wild-goose chase like this. Finally we found one and brought it back to him triumphantly. He was sleeping and so we gave it to his parents.

Matt's father gave us a medical update. The daily blood counts didn't yet show that the transplant was engrafting. Typically the white blood cells recover first, but Matt's counts were still zero. Every morning the oncologist would enter the room and give the number; this was the daily moment of hope and anticipation, yet the news thus far was depressing. It was going to take time, the doctor had said. Matt would have to hang on a little longer than usual.

The day the white cells return is called "breakout day." When neutrophils reach a concentration of five hundred cells per cubic milliliter of blood, Matt would be considered safe from opportunistic infections and would be able to leave his bubble. To commemorate the breakout, the nurses build a large wall outside the bubble using cardboard bricks and streamers. Then the signal is given and the child bursts through the wall and into the hallway. At the entrance to the bone marrow transplant unit hung several Polaroids of children caught at the moment of liberation, Lazarus-like, emerging with wide smiles. Matt just couldn't wait, said his father, for breakout.

Once the white cells returned, though, another problem might arise. Our cells identify themselves using coded proteins on the surface. Discovered in 1958 by the French researcher Jean Dausset these proteins, called human leukocyte antigens or HLA, act as passwords on every one of our cells. While white cells patrol the body, they constantly contact the HLA markers of nearby cells. If the contacted cell fails to present the correct HLA molecule, the white cell strafes the offending cell with powerful destructive enzymes, blasting holes in its membrane and killing it. This is the fundamental principle of the immune system: "self" is tolerated while "non-self" is destroyed. Most commonly this defense system destroys cells that have been infected by viruses, since cells infected by viruses ingeniously alter the HLA on their surfaces. With every kill the immune system becomes more sensitized to particular "non-self" cells and intensifies its attacks. (That's how immunization works. One introduces a small amount of a foreign material in the body—like giving an attack dog a suspect's scent—which whips the immune system into frenzy. Even years later, the slightest invasion by the foreign material prompts a counterattack so precise and so thorough that the infection is eliminated without the host's awareness.)

Unfortunately, the cells that protected Matt's father so loyally didn't anticipate being placed into another body. Each of us has six types of HLA, and our white cells are used to them. When placed in a foreign person with different HLA, the cells go berserk, destroying everything around them like well-armed combatants dropped onto a beachhead of enemies. This is known as graft versus host disease. This is the opposite problem faced by people who receive organ transplants like kidneys or livers. The host's immune cells attack the new organ, a situation called "rejection."

To minimize the risk of graft versus host disease, Matt's oncologist tested all of Matt's family for their complement of HLA types. Matt's father was the closest match, at five of six HLA being identical. Since a perfect match—six out of six—would be better, Matt's doctors also searched for unrelated potential donors through a national registry.

No national registry existed until 1977, when a ten-year-old girl named Laura Graves was diagnosed with leukemia in Fort Collins, Colorado, and referred to the Fred Hutchinson Cancer Research Center in Seattle for a bone marrow transplant. Before then, the only transplants ever done were between identical twins or perfectly matched family members. Unfortunately, Laura had no suitable match among her family members, as only 30 percent of people have a match within their family. At Seattle, a frantic search of HLA types was undertaken among regular blood product donors.

Incredibly, an identical match was found in a staff member who worked in the hospital laboratory. The odds of a perfect match in an unrelated person are about one in twenty thousand, so Laura was lucky indeed. The recipient of the world's first unrelated marrow transplant, Laura successfully engrafted and had no graft versus host disease.

Laura's father worked tirelessly to organize a national registry, which began operation in 1987 and facilitated its first transplant within one year. Still, many children like Matt fail to find donors through national registries. In 1995, the parents of six-year-old Molly Nash were unable to find a match for their daughter. Molly desperately needed marrow for a rare genetic blood disease called Fanconi anemia that was further complicated by leukemia. With help from geneticist Charles Strom, the parents decided to have another baby: a test tube baby specifically selected to have HLA identical to Molly's. After five miscarriages, the couple succeeded, and the blood from the placenta of Molly's new brother (so-called cord blood, which is rich in stem cells) was transplanted immediately. It was a success and Molly is still alive today. While heroic in its way, this strategy clearly isn't for everyone. Given the lack of a perfect match in registries, Matt's best shot had been getting marrow from his father.

Two weeks passed before I saw Matt again. I heard things were not going well. The marrow didn't seem to be engrafting, despite the use of additional medicines called stimulating factors that promote bone marrow growth. Worse, Matt had developed a high fever and a progressive infection. His parents were already losing hope and then Matt slipped into a semicomatose state. That indicated the infection had likely reached his brain and caused meningitis. With no armies of white cells to defend him, Matt depended wholly on the antibiotics he got from his doctors. But there's no substitute for natural immunity, and Matt got worse. He began slipping away.

Again I scrubbed and gowned to enter the bubble. Matt had gotten even paler and thinner, and looked asleep. The alligator basin was gone. Though quite ill, he hadn't yet needed to be placed on a breathing machine. "Hi, Matt," I said to him. He didn't answer. His mother gently told me he hadn't spoken for a few days. His counts hadn't come back up, and now his blood was infected with fungi called *Candida* and bacteria called *Staphylococci*. A continuous infusion of morphine kept him comfortable. Because he had a tendency to thrash his limbs occasionally, his arms were secured to the side of the hospital bed, as were his feet. Like stigmata, bruises lined his wrists and ankles where attempts had been made to draw blood from his arteries.

I stayed a short while and talked with Matt's parents. Just before leaving, I reached out and touched Matt's hand. "See you later," I said, and turned to go. Hearing a rustle behind me, I turned and heard a single word issue from Matt's mouth: "Darshak," my name. It was frankly miraculous that from the residue of electrical impulses that fired less and less purposefully in Matt's infected brain, a word was issued. Somehow a voice processed in his auditory cortex was forwarded to the memory center in his brain's hippocampus, interpreted by the language center, and finally dispatched to the motor area to order my name spoken. As unexpectedly as Matt spoke, he again sank into unconsciousness. Though I'll never know what he meant by saying my name, I think that even in his time of greatest peril, *he* tried to comfort *me*.

The infection proved unstoppable. The same organisms that had once peacefully colonized Matt's skin and mouth ran amok despite the doctors' best efforts and betrayed their host. A few days later, Matt died.

Every year a tree-planting ceremony is held at Camp Sunrise, and the children and staff commemorate previous campers who passed away. We're invited to make small decorations that are hung on the tree's pine branches after the planting. I always make an ornament for Matt in the shape of a butterfly, cutting the pattern with special care from a stenciled piece of orange cardboard. Most years I don't write anything on it, and I'm the only one who knows for whom it is made.

~ 4 ~

Bones

ON THE INTERPRETATION OF OMENS

I

Several years ago, my mother walked down the stairs into the living room and lost her footing. Stumbling, she reached out to grasp the railing with her right hand and came down heavily on her right foot, which twisted inward. Seated nearby, my father heard a sharp crack.

The most frequently injured joint of the body, the ankle is most vulnerable during extension, as when stepping downward. Two long bones, the tibia and the relatively smaller fibula, span the distance from the knee to the ankle, where they are anchored to the foot by powerful cables called ligaments. When my mother landed on her inwardly twisted right foot, the ligament attached to her fibula—the bone on the outside of an ankle—was violently stretched. Because any structure gives way at its weakest point, the thin fibula fractured. This was confirmed at the hospital, and an orthopedic surgeon placed a cast on the foot.

Later, my father said he felt unusually short of breath after carrying my mother to the car on the way to the hospital. It was as though the cracking sound of her skeleton passed to him acoustically and also ethereally, conveying to him not only the immediate knowledge of his wife's injury but a deeper, more sinister affliction. It was the first sign of the great troubles to come.

The term *skeleton* implies potential that must be fleshed out. A skeleton provides the broad suggestions of structure; for example, a skeleton key is filed down to open many locks, a skeleton outline must be filled with detailed content, and a skeleton proof has only the lightest etching, which must be deepened before printmaking.

Human skeletons furnish the outlines of our bodies, the firm scaffolding on which flesh hangs. For solid substances, however, bones have amorphous beginnings. In the uterus, developing babies have bones that are mostly made of cartilage, the rubbery material of earlobes and noses. In growing children, liquid crystals of calcium within this cartilage transform into a solid matrix, just as water freezes into ice, a process called "mineralization," which continues until adolescence. That's how babies' bones eventually harden. To dramatize the importance of these crystals, an interesting experiment is to place an adult chicken bone, which has a structure similar to human bone, in a cup of vinegar for a week. The bone becomes as pliable as an eraser, since vinegar dissolves the calcium.

In addition to mineralizing, a child's bones also grow broader and longer. Like a tree trunk, a child's bone grows circumferentially as its barklike covering (called periosteum) lays down fresh bone. So-called long bones, like those of the legs and arms, lengthen as their expanding ends, or "growth plates," deposit cartilage and calcium on existing bone. The process is gradual but consistent, following a pace similar to the migration of glaciers.

Like the bones of a developing child, the cases in this chapter are initially soft outlines that gradually ossify and grow into directed narratives. As with my mother's broken foot, which first unveiled my father's deadly lung disease, illnesses of bone also serve as omens for other hidden, systemic problems, such as prejudice, superstition, deficiencies in health policy and the legal system, and violence to children.

My father's younger sister, Teeru, cost my grandfather an extra ten thousand rupees to marry off because she was born with six fingers on her left hand. The extra phalanx grew off the middle of her pinky, and the whole appendage resembled the number four. According to my grandfather, a malevolent spirit assaulted Teeru when she was in the womb.

Indian children are immersed in myths regarding evil spirits. During my childhood, my mother painted my eyelids with a black pigment to scare the evil spirits away. As a youth herself she was forbidden from going out alone, lest someone place a hex, or nazar, on her waist-length hair. During pregnancy she took additional precautions, since everyone knew that a pregnant woman was an easy target for evil mischief.

Because she already had a deformity, Teeru was considered to be in great peril during pregnancy. While the additional dowry had certainly persuaded Teeru's husband to overlook some of his wife's poor karma, he hadn't abandoned all of his reservations. He summoned a respected astrologer to determine his unborn child's horoscope. On the seer's counsel, he insisted that Teeru increase her intake of almonds, rice, and spinach. In the final month of gestation, Teeru was forbidden to leave her house, except to visit a temple.

When Teeru's son Jayesh was born, the obstetrician noticed a strawberrylike protrusion at the base of the newborn's back. A thin, transparent layer of skin covered a reddish mass there. When the baby was handed to Teeru, she held him tightly as her husband glared accusingly.

The attitude of Teeru's husband was typical for a conservative man of the time who saw medical complications not as the result of statistical realities but as repayment for immoral acts. My father's family members were conservative Jains who believed in the primacy of nonviolence and forbid even the eating of roots such as onions and garlic, since their consumption required uprooting a plant. Perhaps Teeru had strayed from these strict dietary prescriptions, or performed another spiritual transgression.

Jayesh's spine, or vertebral column, was defective. The protrusion on the newborn's back was a portion of his spinal cord, a condition known as spina bifida. The child's problem began only three weeks after his conception. During that time, he was an oblong ball of cells slightly larger than a grain of rice. In normal development, a lengthwise groove appears on the surface of the embryo. This valley will become the spinal column. At the midpoint of its length, the opposite sides of the groove pinch together, so the embryo resembles a bow tie. Around the twenty-sixth day of development, half of the groove closes, like a zipper, from the midpoint of the embryo's back up to the head. At twenty-nine days, the other half closes in the same manner from the midpoint of the back down to the embryo's rear end. Thus, a small tunnel, called the neural tube, is created.

When the top of the tube fails to zip shut, the brain has no vault in which to develop and anencephaly—literally, "no brain"—occurs. Half of these children die in the womb. The rest usually expire shortly after birth. If only a portion of the top of the neural tube closes, part of the brain protrudes from the skull, a devastating problem called encephalocoele. Most of these children also die, and those who survive are severely retarded.

Jayesh had a problem with the other end of the neural tube. When the bottom of the tube remains open, the spinal bones or vertebrae do not form properly. This is why part of his spinal cord was exposed. Teeru recalled how a neurosurgeon saw Jayesh and was relieved that the infant could move his legs. That meant the vertebral defect spared the nerves of the legs. However, Jayesh needed surgery to cover the remains of the cord.

I first met Jayesh and his mother in my grandfather's Bombay apartment when I was six years old, and Jayesh was four. Teeru was a remarkably good-humored woman who had bought us some soda called Thums-Up and told outrageous tall tales about her extra finger. Every few hours, she walked Jayesh to the parlor's corner where there was a small drain. There, Jayesh pulled off his shorts and Teeru depressed his belly. Later, I learned this was a medical maneuver called a *credé*. In this manner, Teeru evacuated Jayesh's bladder periodically because the child was unable to urinate voluntarily. The rest of the family continued about their business, paying no mind. As I grew older, though, I sometimes heard my aunts speculating about what Teeru might have done to deserve a "defective" child.

In the same city where Jayesh lived, Lucy Wills in 1931 had begun work that would eventually absolve Teeru of any responsibility for her son's condition. Wills was interested in a curious form of anemia that affected pregnant women. Twelve years earlier, physician William Osler noted that this problem, "pernicious anemia of pregnancy," occurred late and spontaneously improved after a baby's delivery, unlike "common pernicious anemia," which affected men and nonpregnant women and was invariably fatal if untreated. Though beef liver was used successfully to cure common pernicious anemia in 1928, Wills discovered its vexing lack of efficacy in pernicious anemia of pregnancy. However, she soon discovered that Marmite, a type of yeast extract, did work.

Wills found that pernicious anemia was caused by two different nutritional deficiencies: one that was corrected by eating beef liver (as in common pernicious anemia) and the other abolished by eating Marmite (as in pernicious anemia of pregnancy). As with many seminal discoveries, the importance of Wills's work was left unrealized for over a decade. In the 1940s, a biochemist at the University of Texas isolated thirty-six milligrams of a new growth factor from a half-ton of spinach, which he named folic acid, after the Latin *folium*, for leaf. In short order, scientists realized that this was the mysterious vitamin found in Marmite that cured pernicious anemia of pregnancy, a condition affecting almost 25 percent of pregnant women. (Of note, common pernicious anemia is caused by a deficiency of vitamin B_{12}, which is copious in beef liver.)

This seemingly obscure blood problem has an important negative impact on bone development. In 1965, an obstetrician reported that almost 70 percent of his patients who delivered children with a neural tube defect, Jayesh's problem, had pernicious anemia of pregnancy. He hypothesized that folate deficiency could cause these birth defects.

He was right. A large trial involving almost two thousand English women was prematurely ended in 1991 when it became clear that folic acid could reduce the number of cases of spina bifida by over 70 percent. Within a year, the U.S. Public Health Service recommended that all women of childbearing age take a daily folic acid supplement.

What then occurred can only be described as a public health failure, a combination of inadequate political will and poor government policy. The prevention of neural tube defects should have galvanized authorities. In the words of Robert Brent, a prominent researcher, "Folic acid–sensitive birth defects are as preventable as polio," yet today hundreds of thousands of children continue to be born with such defects. Brent notes that every year in the United States there are more children born with preventable neural tube defects than the total number of thalidomide-deformed babies born in all of Europe, including those from the height of the crisis there. What happened?

The problem is that—at least in the United States—almost half of all pregnancies are unplanned. Few women follow the recommendation to take a daily folate supplement for most of their lives. Additionally, many women believe that a daily pill is a hassle if they're not trying to conceive; they start taking folate upon learning they're pregnant. Unfortunately, the neural tube and vertebral column usually is formed before then.

Recently, in South Carolina, a well-funded campaign to educate women about the efficacy of preconception folic acid increased its use from 8 percent to 30 percent of eligible women, which was still inadequate. Since then, folate has been added to flour, a key food staple. This strategy follows similar approaches to prevent thyroid goiter (by adding iodine to salt), cavities (by adding fluoride to water), and rickets (by adding vitamin D to milk). In 1996, the U.S. Food and Drug Administration ordered that all enriched grain products be fortified with folate within two years.

Unfortunately, the dosage is too small to be effective. Against the recommendations of the March of Dimes, the American Academy of Pediatrics, and the U.S. Centers for Disease Control, the FDA required only 140 micrograms of folate per 100 grams of flour instead of 350 micrograms. On average, the proportion of women consuming enough folate to prevent neural tube defects (400 micrograms daily) increased by only 3 percent.

The FDA chose reduced supplementation for an unusual reason. Though folate is safe even in large amounts—up to twenty-five times the recommended daily dose—large doses might also help (for complex biochemical reasons) common pernicious anemia due to vitamin B_{12} deficiency. While the anemia of these people theoretically might improve, other problems such as dementia and spinal cord problems, which are also caused by vitamin B_{12} deficiency, continue. The FDA argued that leaving such individuals anemic was critical so that they might—presumably due to symptoms of anemia, such as fatigue or passing out—come to the attention of a doctor and get treated with vitamin B_{12}, which would also help the dementia and nerve damage. The FDA believed excessive folate fortification of flour would mask common pernicious anemia, which affects almost 1 percent of the elderly, and cause an outbreak of neurological problems.

The FDA was worried about unintended consequences, a variant of the "butterfly effect," described in detail by James Gleick in his book *Chaos*, in which a butterfly flapping its wings in Beijing might eventually cause a storm in New York. Certainly public health authorities have been burned before; for example, a surprise outbreak of an acute paralysis called Guillain-Barré syndrome followed large-scale swine flu vaccination in the 1970s. Adding the appropriate amount of folic acid to flour seemed to be too big a public health gamble.

But data supporting this concern are lacking. A comprehensive search of Medline, a database of all published medical articles, fails to locate a single case of pernicious anemia missed as a result of folic acid supplementation at the dose needed to prevent neural tube defects. In a 1989 national survey of almost one thousand practicing blood specialists, researchers were also unable to find a single doctor who reported finding such a case. The FDA's concerns appear wholly theoretical. In any event, many nutritionists have pointed out that a strategy of adding *both* vitamin B_{12} and folate to flour would obviate any possibility of masking pernicious anemia, but this proposal hasn't yet received serious consideration.

Still, the discovery of folate's role in preventing neural tube defects is a reassuring parable, in which a slowly solidifying body of medical knowledge replaces superstition and blame. A few years ago, my cousin Jayesh (who still uses credés to empty his bladder) married in a traditional Jain ceremony, arriving on a white horse to meet his bride. On the wedding dais, Jayesh garlanded his wife and they circled the sacred marriage fire seven times, receiving blessings from the priest each time. My uncle's attitude toward my aunt's imaginary misdeeds seemed to soften with time, and on that day he and Teeru sat just to the left of the dais during the ceremony, holding hands. Though his parents still consult an astrologer for *rashis*, Jayesh considers the resulting recommendations a cultural entertainment and not a true prescription. And though his children have a slightly increased risk for having a neural tube defect, Jayesh sees this not as a karmic burden but merely a biochemical one.

Nick Flamel loved to climb trees. The seven-year-old was a wizard at finding the right knots on a trunk, and balancing just so on them to scamper up to the next branch. But on the day we met, his instincts failed. He fell ten feet. Nick landed on his outstretched hands and felt immediate, searing pain.

In the emergency room, the triage nurse noted Nick's swollen left forearm and sent him to the radiology suite for X rays. (To save time, triage nurses often obtain lab tests or X rays before a doctor sees a patient.) There, the X rays of various action figures and household items that lined the waiting room delighted Nick. A technician called Nick and took several X rays of the boy's arm in various orientations. These methods have changed little since 1896, when the first medical X ray taken in North America demonstrated that a teenage boy had broken his wrist while ice-skating. After developing Nick's films, the technician directed the family back to the emergency room to see me.

It was a busy day in the fall, and the ER was crammed with patients. I hastily blew my nose—almost all of the doctors were sick with something or other, as we were continuously inoculated with various illnesses from our patients—and reviewed Nick's chart outside his room. I knocked and entered.

Nick was a bright-eyed, red-haired boy who cradled his left arm in some discomfort. "Tell him what happened," said Mr. Flamel. Nick sheepishly explained he was trying to follow his cat up the tree when he lost his footing. "I saw it happen," added Nick's mother. "He didn't hit his head, and he didn't pass out or vomit or have a seizure. He just hit the grass with his arms and started crying." That was reassuring; Nick was at much less risk for a paralyzing neck fracture or head bleed.

I examined Nick's head and neck. There were no bruises or tender spots, confirming that it was unnecessary to obtain skull or neck X rays. I held Nick's right arm and performed a series of maneuvers to test his bones and muscles, which were all normal. I repeated the tests on his left arm. He had an exquisitely tender red swelling just before his wrist. Despite the pain, Nick had no problem moving his fingers and wrist, which meant the fall hadn't injured any nerves. "What kind of cat do you have?" I asked while checking the legs and feet for pain. Nick answered, "Black." After the exam, I went to review the X rays at the light-box near the nurses' station.

X rays are critical since there's no other way to see bones. But why are bones hidden in the inside of the body? The answer is best understood from an evolutionary perspective. Without internal bones, locomotion on land would be physically impossible for humans. Purposeful movement first evolved in plants, like the shy mimosa that retracts its leaves on touch, or any of the hundreds of plants whose leaves open and close in a regular fashion during the day. These plants have no bones or muscles; instead, certain specialized cells rapidly release water and deflate like balloons, causing the leaves to move. Called "turgor-pressure change," this strategy generates only small forces that can't support locomotion. Hence, primitive animals evolved muscle cells. In earthworms, for example, these fibers are arranged in two planes: circular bands around the worm (which lengthen the worm during contraction) and longitudinal bands down its length (which shorten the worm). The circular bands contract first to push part of the worm forward. Then the longitudinal bands contract and pull along the rest of the body.

Still, worms lack a skeleton and can't develop advanced forms of locomotion like walking. Arthropods like crabs developed hard outer-body coverings called exoskeletons that contain their muscles and organs. This additional support allowed the animals to grow more complex and also provided a protective shield from predators. However, exoskeletons impose limitations on an animal's size. Large animals require exoskeletons that are far too heavy to be practical on land. All substantial animals with exoskeletons, such as king crabs and lobsters, are aquatic, since the buoyancy of water provides support that their weight demands. Thus, endoskeletons—the bones we all have—evolved. Our internal bones are stronger than exoskeletons and do not confine our muscles, which are of sufficient size to support our larger bodies.

I located Nick's X rays. One of the two long bones of the forearm, the ulna, was broken all the way through at its midpoint. The child needed a cast. Though the fracture was quite obvious on the first film, it was imperceptible on another taken at a slightly different angle. An old radiology aphorism declares, "One view is no view," and these films illustrated the point well. Since a fracture occurs in a three-dimensional space, a single X ray can appear misleadingly normal. Suppose one takes a broomstick, breaks it in half, and then holds the ends together again. Now assume one hand is held out slightly farther than the other. From the front, an observer might think that the broomstick was whole, whereas a view from above would clearly show that the broomstick was in two pieces. The same confusion can occur with fractures, so they're always evaluated by at least two X rays.

The second radiology saying for broken bones is, "One above and one below." Joints near a fracture are at risk of injury and should also be filmed. Giovanni Monteggia, who described dislocations of the elbow associated with fractures of the ulna, had appreciated this lesson in 1814. So Nick's wrist and elbow were also X rayed, and they looked okay to me.

I paged the orthopedic surgeon on call, who happened to be my former medical school roommate, Tom Marble. He looked almost broken himself when he arrived, weakened by a monthlong regimen of "q twos." In medical lingo, the letter q designates an interval. Therefore the designation "q 4h" that follows Tylenol orders means the drug is taken every four hours, and daily medications like aspirin are designated "q day." Residents refer to the frequency of their calls, or overnight shifts, in the same way. At my training program, pediatric residents take "q fours," staying overnight every fourth night. That means I got a single Saturday and Sunday in a row off per month, and like every pediatric resident, I looked forward hungrily to the monthly "golden weekend." But Tom had to withstand a more punishing schedule; he worked "q twos," or consecutive thirty-six-hour shifts separated by only twelve-hour breaks.

Reviewing the X rays, Tom pointed out that the two ends of the fractured ulna were not lined up perfectly. Nick would need a "reduction," a fairly primitive procedure where one sedates a child with nitrous oxide, "laughing gas" (which is poorly named—a more descriptive name would be "amnesia air" since the child still screams during the procedure but then simply forgets about it), and wrenches a limb until the bones align properly. I introduced Tom to Nick and his family, and Tom escorted them to the orthopedic procedure room for the reduction. As I sat at the physician station completing Nick's chart note, horrifying screams emerged from the procedure room. A few minutes later, Tom opened the door and Nick walked out smiling, already oblivious to his ordeal. A purple fiberglass cast covered Nick's arm.

Rather than healing a bone, a cast only immobilizes it to prevent further injury. Like the mythological phoenix, bone then remakes itself from its remains. In a healthy person, a skeleton is continuously broken down and remade. Before a child reaches one year of age every one of his 206 bones has been "remodeled"; this pace slows somewhat, but an adult still replaces 10 to 20 percent of the skeleton yearly. Inside us, cells called osteoclasts behave like Pac-Men and continuously gobble away bone. Their companions, the osteoblasts, trail immediately and lay new crystals of calcium hydroxyapatite, the scaffolding of bone. We are all, in a sense, under construction. (In older women, shifting hormone levels imbalance this process, causing osteoporosis.)

Fractures are temporary. Osteoblasts and osteoclasts erase the break bit by bit over a few weeks. After a few months, even X rays may fail to show any injury. If, however, the bones are misaligned in a cast the bone may heal with a permanent deformity, which requires intentional rebreaking and recasting by an orthopedic surgeon. That's why a good reduction is so important.

Before discharging Nick, I gave him a follow-up appointment for a cast check in a few weeks. I signed his cast with a black marker and wished him luck. "Did you know today is the first of the month?" Nick asked. No, I answered, and then asked why he mentioned it. "I forgot to say 'Rabbit rabbit,'" explained Nick, "and look what happened."

II

In the spring of 1997, a baby's fractures and other injuries convinced several physicians at my hospital that a crime had taken place. In the sensational trial that followed, the child's broken skeleton became a scaffold for a complicated, contentious debate about whether pediatricians could accurately diagnose intentional injury. Though child abuse as a clinical entity had gradually ossified over decades from a nebulous, poorly defined diagnosis into a solid one (largely due to the work of certain courageous radiologists), the case demonstrated how easily this development could be reversed, like soaking a bone in vinegar.

The emergency department at Children's Hospital has thirty-one rooms numbered by colored signs, and each color implies a severity of illness. The red and black areas, comprising ten rooms, are used for routine complaints such as infant fever, mild dehydration, and various aches and pains. The green section is reserved for more acute cases, including asthma attacks or severe abdominal pain. The blue area, taking its name from the feared "code blue" denoting cardiac or respiratory arrest, has two trauma bays reserved for the direst emergencies, such as high-speed motor accidents. On February 4, 1997, eight-month-old Matthew Eappen was rushed into a blue bay with respiratory arrest of unknown cause.

At 3:46 P.M. that day, a 911 dispatch operator received a frantic call from Louise Woodward, an eighteen-year-old British au pair who looked after Matthew and his two-year-old brother Brendan when their parents were at work. Woodward reported she had found Matthew suddenly unresponsive. "Help! There's a baby. He's barely breathing! He's not focusing his eyes. Help, help, what should I do?" she cried, according to courtroom transcripts. The dispatcher directed two paramedics immediately to the Eappens' house, where they arrived three minutes later. They found a comatose child on the floor, with a stable heartbeat but very shallow, slow breathing. Ashen-faced and critically ill, Matthew held his arms stiffly to his sides, in an involuntary reflex that indicates severe brain damage. Immediately, the paramedics launched into a procedure that was itself reflexive: establish an open airway, then assist breathing, then ensure proper circulation. A pulse oximeter, a device that measures oxygen by beaming a red light through skin, was placed on Matthew's finger and confirmed that he was breathing inadequately. The paramedics placed a small plastic mask over Matthew's face and blew pure oxygen into his lungs with squeezes of an inflatable bag, loaded Matthew into their ambulance, and began the short drive to the emergency room. En route, they made a "10-minute out" call to Children's Hospital and spoke with Ken Mandl, a lanky, energetic doctor who alerted his code team to assemble.

A flurry of activity precedes the arrival of any critically ill child to a blue bay. Mandl strategically placed his code team around the aseptic fifteen-by-twenty-foot room. Three nurses drew resuscitation medications into syringes to be immediately injected if needed, and a radiology technician with a portable X-ray unit and two respiratory therapists were paged. David Greenes was assigned to the head of the bay and prepared to control the infant's breathing, and two residents stood at his sides and readied intravenous catheters. Mandl, the most senior doctor and therefore the "code leader," stood detached several feet from the others to orchestrate the entire process. Once everyone was in position, Mandl pondered the situation in the brief lull. Children rarely become so sick so quickly, he knew, and the list of possible causes was not long. The team would first consider and treat possible seizures, overwhelming infection, cardiac failure, and unusual problems with body electrolytes.

At 4:07 P.M., Matthew arrived and was immediately covered by gloved hands. Within five minutes, monitoring equipment was affixed to his chest, intravenous lines were inserted into his arm and foot, a urinary catheter was inserted into his bladder, a protective collar was applied to his neck, and a breathing tube was passed through his mouth into his trachea. After sending blood for testing, Mandl ordered the administration of antibiotics and antiseizure agents. He was still puzzled. "Nobody knew exactly what was going on," he said.

From the house, Louise Woodward had paged the Eappens with the news that Matthew had been taken to the emergency room. Sunil Eappen, an anesthesiologist at the adjacent Brigham and Women's Hospital, arrived out of breath and still wearing surgical scrubs. Deborah Eappen, who worked farther away, came soon afterward. Stricken, they helplessly watched as the doctors and nurses worked on Matthew. Following standard practice in evaluating coma of unknown cause, Mandl decided to order a computed tomogram (CT) scan of Matthew's head. Just before sending the child to the radiology suite, Mandl bent cheek to cheek with his patient and peered into the pupils with a handheld ophthalmoscope. Dismayed, he saw a sea of crimson instead of the usual orderly lattice of blood vessels. He was looking at a retinal hemorrhage.

The retina is a tissue-thin layer of nerves and blood vessels at the rear of the eye. Though delicate, it generally resists injury better than the blood vessels of the brain. Mandl therefore realized that the retinal hemorrhages almost certainly meant brain bleeding, which explained why Matthew was so critically ill. Paradoxically, the skull that so effectively protects the brain also makes it extremely vulnerable to certain kinds of injuries. Because the brain occupies a closed space that cannot expand, enough excess material like blood in the same space can cause fatal compression of the brain. "We all knew a retinal bleed was a likely death sentence," Mandl recalled. He quickly paged the resident ophthalmologist to confirm the eye findings before Matthew went to the CT scanner.

Before the resident arrived, though, the team learned that Deborah Eappen also was an ophthalmologist. As they waited, Gary Fleischer, another senior physician, gently explained to her why, of the multiple specialists available at Children's Hospital, Mandl had selected an ophthalmologist to see Matthew urgently. Deborah Eappen was so taken aback by the possibility of retinal bleeding that after the resident arrived and completed an exam, she borrowed the glass examination lenses from the resident. As the previously bustling room plunged into silence, she looked carefully into her comatose son's eyes. There was no doubt: the hemorrhages were present, and the full horror of Matthew's prognosis flooded her.

"I knew what that meant," she later said. "I was shocked. I couldn't believe it."

Had this situation occurred a few decades earlier, only one physician in the United States, a radiologist named John Caffey, would have known the most likely cause of Matthew's brain bleed. The cause of hemorrhage inside the skull, or intracranial bleeding, had been a long-debated and poorly understood phenomenon in infants, and Caffey thought he finally understood its origin. In 1946, he published the abstruse-sounding "Multiple fractures in the long bones of infants suffering from chronic subdural hematoma" in the *American Journal of Roentgenology*. Caffey's paper ended many years of speculation about the origin of intracranial bleeds in children.

The dubious nature of these bleeds was described as early as A.D. 200 in the textbook of the Greek obstetrician Soranus. Realizing that an overly stressed caregiver could be dangerous, he made a fascinating observation that foreshadowed Caffey's discovery. Soranus advised new mothers to be careful in selecting a wet nurse, for those without "an even temperament" would let babies "shake and tremble [and] come back with large heads and water on the brain," the earliest known description of probable intracranial bleeding.

The first physician to study infant brain bleeds systematically, the nineteenth-century German pathologist Rudolph Virchow, thought they were just due to infection. Virchow knew that the meninges, the three-layered membranes covering the brain, serve as a scaffold for blood vessels supplying the brain. He thought that "meningitis," or infection of the meninges, caused these blood vessels to bleed. Because the blood was often found under the outermost layer of the meninges, the dura, the type of bleeding Virchow described was called subdural bleeding. This illness seemed to be common. In 1890, the German pathologist Doehle performed four hundred autopsies on children and found that almost one-tenth had subdural bleeds, also thought to be caused by infection.

About a half-century later, in the same hospital where Matthew Eappen would be treated, David Sherwood in 1930 began to speculate that such bleeds might be influenced by a child's home environment. His approach was unique because he inquired about the children's living conditions. The histories were striking: half his

cases were from "dubious home conditions," including a malnourished child of a neglectful mother, and numerous children in foster
homes or institutions. However, Sherwood stopped short of infer-
ring intentional battery, instead stating that the "etiology is obscure."

In his famous 1946 paper, Caffey finally mustered enough confidence to say what no one else did: only traumatic injury could
explain many brain bleeds. A radiologist who read X rays but didn't
often interview patients, Caffey described six children who had subdural bleeding in association with multiple other skeletal fractures
and a suspicious history from caregivers. By associating long bone
fractures with subdural bleeding in these cases, Caffey clearly showed
that the children sustained forceful injury, and he became the
first American physician to suggest that serious trauma was causing infant brain bleeds. Although he didn't directly state that the
injuries were purposefully inflicted, he wrote, "The causal relationship between the traumatic force and damage to the bone is clear. It
is unlikely that trivial unrecognized trauma caused the fractures."

Over the next several years, Caffey become convinced that many
such injuries were intentional, and broadcast his theory with mes-
sianic zeal. In one of his more forcefully worded papers, he insisted
that a radiologist "must stand his ground after his own diagnosis of
trauma and urge his trauma-insensitive colleagues to go into the
history more fully." One can imagine him sitting in his darkened,
quiet reading room perusing X rays day after day, wondering why
the repetitive injuries so obvious to him were so opaque to the primary physicians. Frustrated, he wrote:

Pediatricians, faced with unexplained pain and swelling in the
extremities, in the absence of a history of injury, customarily set
out on an elaborate search for lesions produced by more sophisti-
cated causal agents such as vitamin deficiencies, metabolic im-
balances, infections, neoplasms, reticuloendothelial proliferations,
prenatal disturbances, and chromosomal injuries contracted in

earlier generations. Simple direct mechanical trauma often receives short shrift by those bent on solving the mysteries of more exotic diseases.

Despite the publication of Caffey's work, medical professionals took little notice of it until sixteen years later, when C. Henry Kempe of Denver, Frederic Silverman of Boston, and three colleagues defined the "battered child syndrome" in the *Journal of the American Medical Association* in 1962. (Occasionally, doctors suspecting battery still coyly write "Rule out Silverman's syndrome" on X-ray orders.) The paper is an unusual scientific document; there is no hypothesis, no detailed methods section, and no experimental data. The authors simply described their experience working with injured children.

In response, a national epidemic was "discovered," and pent-up denial of child battery exploded. Frederic Silverman, who was Caffey's first trainee and protégé, speculated that the paper was a marketing coup, which franchised the concept of intentional injury by naming it well. (He called it an illustration of "the role of terminology in the propagation of concepts.") The number of published studies about skeletal trauma in children skyrocketed from less than two per year before 1962 to over thirty-five in 1964 and to several hundred a decade later. Radiologists also described other obvious indicators of intentional injury; Paul Kleinman's classic textbook on child abuse reproduced X rays of an open safety pin and light-bulb in a battered infant's rectum, and seven sewing needles impaled in an eleven-year-old boy with belly pain. The ensuing national outcry led to a profusion of laws and agencies at national, state, and local levels. By 1967, every state had passed mandated reporting laws, requiring certain professionals to report all suspected child abuse to authorities. In 1974, Richard Nixon signed the Child Abuse Prevention and Treatment Act, creating a national center providing funding and technical assistance for child abuse services to local governments.

In retrospect, it seems perplexing that child battery was over-looked for so long. Its denial wasn't rooted in a lack of publicity. In 1873, for example, the Catholic missionary Etta Wheeler discovered a severely beaten child named Mary Ellen Wilson living in a New York tenement. City officials ignored Wheeler's repeated overtures for assistance until, of all agencies, the Society for Prevention of Cruelty to Animals became involved. In the torrent of sensational publicity that followed, the Society for Prevention of Cruelty to Children, Save the Children, Newsboy Refugees, and other organi-zations were founded. However, these groups focused not on child battery but on child labor in factories (though Mary Ellen Wilson had never worked in a factory). In the prevailing social climate, child labor was an attractive target for reform since it smacked of slavery, which was intolerable. Although advocacy groups were willing to reform public cruelty to children by investigating and exposing sweatshops, none was willing to fight private cruelty to children in the homes of abusive parents and caretakers.

The recognition of child battery was therefore left to the medical profession, which had its own cadence. In dealing with illness, doc-tors have a near religious reliance on the collective body of pub-lished medical articles, referred to as "the literature." It is therefore conceivable that the lack of any naming of intentional child battery in the literature before 1962 meant that child battery simply didn't exist as a medical entity. But why was the phenomenon not de-scribed in the literature for so long? A pediatrician has an unusual therapeutic relationship with a child, since parents or other care-givers control the patient's contact with the medical system. In pedi-atric care, therefore, an alliance between caregiver and doctor is critical. To accuse a parent of intentional battery would destroy that bond, and with it any hope of continuing to care for a child at risk. Perhaps doctors as a group acted like battered partners; given that they could not endure separation, they simply stayed quiet and hoped they could reform abusers with coaxing and cajoling.

~~~

Like many fledgling pediatricians, I almost missed my first case of intentional injury. A few weeks into my residency, I was seeing patients in the black and red areas of the Children's Hospital emergency room, reserved for common, usually benign conditions. I wrote my name in dry-erase marker on the large patient board, assigning myself the case, and walked over to the room where the child named Tim and his father waited. The triage nurse had listed the eleven-week-old's chief complaint as fever. I knocked on the door and entered.

"Tim's mother couldn't make it," explained the boy's father, a stocky man dressed in a shirt and tie, who sat in a chair and tried to bottle-feed an infant positioned awkwardly in his lap. "She said Tim's been irritable all day, won't be quiet. He's been hot," he added. I pulled up a chair next to Tim's father and launched into the standard interview. After all, fever was probably the most common complaint seen in the emergency room, and I had seen many similar infants earlier. Nothing out of the ordinary came up, and a brief physical exam was normal. "We'll do a few blood tests, a urine test, and we'll need to obtain a small amount of spinal fluid," I said, and he agreed without protest. Spinal taps often spooked parents, but he acceded. "Whatever you have to do, Doc." His deference was flattering, especially to a first-year resident like myself. Leaving the father, a nurse and I took Tim to a procedure room, where we prepped Tim for a spinal tap by holding him naked on his side and cleaning his back with a brown antiseptic. I briefly noted a curved red mark on his buttock. The spinal tap went smoothly, but the nurse commented that Tim seemed upset when his legs were held.

We decided to obtain an X ray of the leg, which showed an unusual "spiral" fracture of the thigh bone, indicating a serious twisting injury. Now I was confused, since only extreme force can break the largest bone in a baby's body. Returning to the examining room, I asked Tim's father if he recalled any falls or injuries Tim could have sustained. He didn't. I sought out the supervising physician for the night, a precise and efficient woman who reviewed the X rays, examined Tim, talked to his father, and then called me outside the room. "Did you see exactly what Tim's father was wearing?" she asked. Not really, I responded, unsure of the question's relevance. "His belt buckle," she explained, with the tone of a doctor diagnosing a simple ear infection. "It's the same shape and pattern as the skin lesion. He might have whipped the kid at some point, maybe broke the leg, too."

I must have looked skeptical, since she explained patiently, "Look, the kid has a spiral fracture, and nothing except twisting can do that. He's only a few months old, so he couldn't have been running and fallen. Someone must have done it, and based on the look of that belt buckle it must be Dad. There's just nothing else that explains the injuries."

The attending advised me to involve the Child Protection Team, which analyzes cases and helps determine if abuse is likely. The CPT social worker helped me alert the state social services department to a case of potential abuse, as required by law. She then reviewed the case with the CPT physician on call and relayed her conclusions to local authorities. The CPT's opinion is weighed heavily by state social services agencies, which ultimately decide where the child will be placed. A child may be sent back to his family without intervention, sent home with regular visitation and support by social workers, or removed from his home. In this case, the state was persuaded by the CPT that Tim would be endangered if sent home, and he was placed in temporary foster care.

A first case of abuse is something of a carnal experience for a resident; it is a frightening, unforgettable, and wholly inevitable step to becoming a mature pediatrician. On a small scale, an intern's first diagnosis of inflicted injury recapitulates the historical acknowledgment of child battery: there is often an initial period of misdirection, a gradually increasing suspicion of the truth, and finally recognition of a problem that in hindsight seems almost obvious.

In addition to a first abuse case, almost every resident at Children's Hospital recalls a lecture by Eli Newberger, the medical director of the CPT. Not long after I saw Tim in the emergency room, Newberger gave my class of residents his annual lecture on recognizing and treating child abuse. Newberger, who founded the CPT in 1970 as a twenty-nine-year-old resident, once told me he "stumbled into the field of child abuse" as an impressionable resident in the 1960s. An internationally recognized jazz musician, Newberger says that his involvement with battered children "connects to the sense of shared struggle and social protest that runs deep in the history and practice of jazz." While he often denied liking the controversy that surrounds his work, I suspected he was secretly attracted to it. Newberger is a man drawn to conflict; for him it is a source of creative energy.

Newberger wanted to make sure that trainees at Children's Hospital would appreciate the breadth and variety of intentional injury. In his lecture, he flipped through slides featuring a disturbing variety of children's injuries, including cigarette and iron burns, scalding by immersion in boiling water, stab wounds, electrocution scars, limbs intentionally bent into unnatural angles, and strangulation. As each slide changed, a murmur of horror went through the audience. Newberger's aim was to expose maltreatment so nakedly that it was undeniable. He continued on to other, more bizarre forms of child battery, including the curious entity of Munchausen syndrome by proxy (MBP). Described originally in the British medical journal *Lancet* in 1977 as the "hinterland of child abuse," MBP usually involves caregivers who secretly inflict injury on children, seek medical care for the problems, and enjoy the subsequent medical and social attention. These cases are bizarre; one involved a mother who periodically injected fecal material into a child's brain, a situation those experienced in the diagnosis of MBP call "stool shooting."

Having evaluated abused children for almost three decades, Newberger long ago stopped being surprised by cases of child battery. He first heard about Matthew Eappen just hours after the child was brought to the emergency room. That afternoon, Ken Mandl communicated his concerns about probable forceful injury to Joanne Michalek, the CPT social worker on call that day. As required by mandatory reporting laws passed in the 1960s, she assisted Mandl in notifying the local department of social services.

Michalek soon learned what transpired after Matthew was taken to radiology and called Newberger at his home. Newberger thought the entire description so convincing for intentional injury that the CPT's involvement seemed almost a formality. He told Michalek, "It sounds like a classic case of abuse. I'll see him in the morning since we're told he's stable enough to make it through the night."

After Ken Mandl confirmed in the emergency room that Matthew had retinal hemorrhages, he sent Matthew to the radiology suite to get a head CT scan. The images showed an immense bleed exerting enough pressure to push Matthew's brain out of position, a critical condition called midline shift. Joseph Madsen, a stocky senior neurosurgeon, was leaving to attend his daughter's music recital when he stopped by the radiology department to glance over an unrelated case. He never made it to the recital. Madsen spied Matthew's CT scan as it came up on a screen and was so dismayed at the amount of bleeding that he rushed Matthew to the operating room. Immediately, Madsen drilled holes into Matthew's head and removed part of the skull to relieve the high pressure. In a child whose brain is under normal pressure, a surgeon opening the skull usually sees only a trickle of fluid. In his remarkable operative report, Madsen described a horrifying explosion of blood:

A small opening in the dura was made and liquid blood squirted out several feet from the patient. [After] the bone fragment was removed the dura was rapidly opened [and] a massive amount of clot extruded itself and delivered from the brain. The brain which was initially pushed down then swelled to beyond its normal dimension. Within another five minutes or so we noticed [the] brain became very firm as it projected like a bread loaf through the cranial defect.

After considering a partial removal of Matthew's brain so that the remainder could be squeezed back into the skull, Madsen instead decided to leave the skull open, in hopes that the brain would return to its normal size. After the surgery, Matthew was admitted to the intensive care unit on life support. All predictors of brain recovery, including eye pupil response to light, spontaneous breathing, and certain reflexive eye movements, were discouraging, even though Matthew's heart and lungs responded well to life support. The next day, the intensive care team obtained a series of X rays, called a skeletal survey, to see if Matthew had any other injuries indicating trauma. He did. The survey showed a skull fracture, which appeared recent, and a wrist fracture, which appeared one to four weeks old (though the radiologist noted that the fractures were difficult to date precisely). A senior ophthalmologist, Lois Smith, examined Matthew's left eye and described "folding" of the retina in addition to the previously noticed bleeding. She described these findings as "pathognomonic" for child abuse, meaning that even if she didn't consider Matthew's brain bleed and fractures, the retina showed irrefutable evidence of sudden, forceful injury of the type usually seen in high-speed car accidents.

Matthew's brain failed to recover and his other organs began to deteriorate. The Eappens held vigil for the next four days. Repeated CT scans showed extensive areas of brain death, and neurologists could not elicit any significant brain function when examining

Matthew. On February 9, Sunil and Deborah Eappen met with Matthew's medical team and were told that the odds of recovery were now so poor that withdrawal of life support should be considered. The Eappens agreed, and sometime after 10 P.M., the baby's ventilator was turned off. Matthew's parents played children's music, lit a candle, and took turns holding him. At 10:57 P.M., Matthew was pronounced dead.

From the outset, suspicion of intentional injury fell on the au pair, Louise Woodward. One hour after bringing Matthew to the emergency room, the paramedics alerted Newton police detective William Byrne to a possible child battery case in his town's jurisdiction. Byrne called Mandl, who told him that Matthew had almost certainly received a forceful blow to the head. Byrne then drove to the Eappens' home to interrogate Woodward, arriving in the evening around the same time Matthew was being admitted to Children's Hospital's intensive care unit after his surgery. Woodward told Byrne she was "a little rough" with Matthew, had "dropped him on some towels in the bathroom," and at one point "delicately shaken him." Byrne asked her to demonstrate with a doll, and Woodward gingerly shook it. Giving Woodward what he called "the benefit of the doubt," Byrne took his leave after asking where she was spending the night, in case he had more questions.

The following morning, Eli Newberger evaluated Matthew and believed he had sustained acute, inflicted injury. "What else could it possibly be?" he rhetorically asked me later. Though the scenario was familiar, even routine, Newberger was still angered. Despite the pity he occasionally feels for batterers, Newberger doesn't believe any circumstance absolves them from personal responsibility. He is motivated by a deep moral outrage and wants them to face punishment. He decided that he had no qualms about testifying against

Woodward, the only caregiver who was with Matthew for the seven hours before the 911 call. "She was guilty," he said to me simply, "and she should be accountable."

The same day, Byrne spoke with Madsen and heard a graphic description of Matthew's injuries. Now more suspicious, Byrne called the home of a coordinator of the agency E. F. Au Pair, where Woodward was staying, to ask more questions. A lawyer answered the phone, and Byrne never spoke to Woodward.

Given the opinions of Mandl and now Madsen, Byrne took Woodward into custody for assault and battery of a child, a charge elevated to murder after Matthew's death. Three weeks later, a grand jury heard key testimony from several physicians including Newberger, who said that Woodward had shaken Matthew so hard that his developing brain "smashed back and forth within his skull" and that the final injury was a "severe traumatic impact against a hard surface." The jury accepted that "extreme cruelty" may have motivated Woodward, and she was indicted for first-degree murder and held without bail. (Massachusetts allows first-degree murder indictments in the absence of premeditation if "cruelty" or "atrocity" is involved.)

Though some of Matthew's doctors expected a quick resolution, the Woodward trial became an international media event. To begin with, the British press was fresh from the funeral of Princess Diana and recently exposed to American trials in the O. J. Simpson prosecution, and Woodward represented a sort of media hybrid of these stories: a virtuous paragon tried by an unfair system. One British tabloid pontificated, "American justice . . . O. J. Simpson is innocent and Louise Woodward is a child-killer." The trial involved a Briton tried in the American court system, and British coverage of the trial had a decidedly sporting flavor; the London *Guardian* commented that the case "may officially be the State of Massachusetts vs. Louise Woodward in that courtroom, but it's also America vs. Britain."

(Without a touch of irony, lawyer Alan Dershowitz also wondered on CNN's *Larry King Live* whether local criticism of Woodward was cultural since Boston's Irish roots created anti-English bias.)

Second, the British and American publics were increasingly skeptical that many allegations of child abuse could be substantiated and were poised to direct anger toward accusers. In 1987, two pediatricians from Cleveland County in Leeds, England, used an endoscopic technique described in a *Lancet* article (provocatively titled "Buggery in Childhood") to diagnose rectal penetration in one hundred twenty children. Many of these children were removed from their homes, without explanation to the children or parents. A media outcry ensued. The seeming arbitrariness of these actions in the so-called Cleveland affair created conspicuous distrust of child protection agencies, and even years later the *Sunday Telegraph* bemoaned "how easily over-officiousness and ignorance can result in innocent parents being falsely prosecuted." In the early 1990s, Americans witnessed the retraction of entire "diseases" involving childhood battery, including satanic ritual abuse, multiple personality disorder, and recovered memory syndrome. In many cases, patients later dubbed their memories of childhood abuse a figment of the imagination and won spectacular multimillion-dollar lawsuits against physicians who encouraged their fantasies.

Last, the case stoked class and ethnic tensions. Sunil and Deborah Eappen, both physicians, lived in an affluent suburb of Boston and were perceived by some people as harsh taskmasters of their au pair; one Boston laborer told *USA Today* that the Eappens "expected Woodward to be a slave." Another columnist wrote that critics believed Woodward "was given too much responsibility by a woman shirking her own." The Eappens were blamed for retaining an ill-motivated, poorly experienced caregiver who frequently missed her curfew and was once caught leaving their children unattended. One radio caller in Boston opined, "She is guilty of manslaughter," referring not to Woodward but to Deborah Eappen. Additionally, the

Eappens are a mixed couple (Sunil Eappen is South Asian; Deborah Eappen is white), and covert racism may have swayed sympathy away from them.

In these circumstances, a courtroom was not the right place to expect a productive dialogue about child battery. The trial became a confusing, often dishonest, medical debate that ultimately led the judge and many observers to conclude that a severe, sudden injury never happened.

Shortly after Woodward's indictment, Massachusetts district attorney Tom Reilly appointed Gerard Leone and Martha Coakley to try the case for the prosecution. For the defense, the agency that placed Woodward with the Eappens, E. F. Au Pair, engaged the Boston firm of Silverglate & Good, who also recommended hiring Barry Scheck, an attorney experienced in forensic medical cases. After several delays, the trial was set to begin in early October, eight months after Matthew's death.

In his 1962 paper, Kempe wrote, "The bones tell a story that the child is too young or too afraid to tell." Since then, the advent of CT scans, nuclear bone imaging, improved recognition of ophthalmologic trauma, and new surgical techniques expanded the tale a child's body can tell. Louise Woodward's trial wasn't only about Matthew's bones, but also about his brain and eyes. The prosecution assembled eight doctors from various Children's Hospital divisions, including emergency, radiology, pathology, neurosurgery, child protection, and ophthalmology, who testified that Matthew's injuries were nonaccidental and acute. Between them, these physicians had evaluated hundreds of injured children and authored an equivalent number of scientific papers. Physicians polled by *U.S. News and World Report* have selected their hospital as the best pediatric facility in the country yearly for over a decade.

At his office overlooking downtown Boston, Leone sat at his

desk, which had a small picture of Matthew Eappen next to pictures of his own children, and later explained the prosecution's strategy to me: "We argued there was simply no sensible explanation for Matthew's injuries other than abuse."

On October 7, 1997, Leone said in an opening statement that Woodward "in a frustrated, resentful, unhappy attitude, slammed the baby into a hard object and shook him, causing his death— actions that anyone would know would result in death. In this Commonwealth, that is murder." Defense counsel Andrew Good countered by telling the jury that defense experts "are going to tell you this was no slamming." He continued, "This child came to the emergency room with absolutely not a mark on him, no external sign of trauma." If Matthew had actually sustained the alleged trauma there should have been "a smashed and destroyed head." What actually happened, Good closed, was that Matthew suffered an earlier injury, possibly from an accident, that resulted in blood leaking into his skull over several weeks.

Matthew's bones told a very clear story. However, almost from the beginning, the prosecution made errors that undermined its case. The first medical witness for the prosecution, emergency physician Ken Mandl, described how Matthew first came to the hospital, and how nothing but forceful injury explained Matthew's bleeds. (Mandl had written in his chart with confidence, "Trauma X physical abuse strongly suspected.") In a tense cross-examination, Scheck confronted Mandl with the previous grand jury testimony of Gerald Feigin, a forensic pathologist who had examined Matthew's brain and said the force needed to cause the observed injury was equivalent to that of "a fifteen-foot fall onto a hard surface." (Neurosurgeon Madsen made a similar statement in his deposition.) Reiterating the comparison, Scheck asked Mandl if there were any bruises or other external findings indicating that Matthew's head had "slammed down onto a hard surface with the force equivalent to dropping a child from a height of fifteen feet onto concrete." Mandl didn't explain that such external injuries are frequently absent even in confessed battery cases, and therefore irrelevant. Instead, he acquiesced, "There were no findings to specifically indicate that, no."

The misleading "fifteen-foot fall" analogy haunted the prosecution's case. It was a mistake to compare Matthew's injury to a fall from a specific height, since this estimate was speculative. This was the first of multiple tactical errors made by the prosecution. Their frustrating lack of a confession, an eyewitness, or medical proof thoroughly convincing to laypersons led them to mistakenly create specific scenarios that could not be substantiated. Analogies are effective explanatory devices because they simplify complex phenomena and are easily recalled. Conversely, they are deadly for the same reasons when retracted. The confusion regarding estimates of times and distances was apparent and damaged the credibility of Matthew's doctors.

Another error was made on the sixth day of testimony when Eli Newberger took the stand. Leone asked him, "Do you have an opinion concerning the manner of infliction of injuries to Matthew's eyes, skull, and brain?" With brisk confidence, Newberger answered, "My opinion is that this child was violently shaken for a prolonged period. This shaking was to such a violent degree that it would have required as much energy as an adult could muster, sustained over a period of time up to or exceeding a minute, possibly delivered in intervals." Newberger then mimed how hard Woodward had to have shaken Matthew to produce a subdural bleed. While dramatic, the demonstration was not entirely accurate, since most child abuse experts agree that shaking alone might not cause skull fractures and subdural bleeds.

Looking back on the trial, several of Matthew's doctors expressed frustrations because they realized Woodward hurt Matthew but were unable to show exactly how. In retrospect, they underestimated the judge and jury's ability to grasp medical concepts; perhaps they should have explained areas of medical uncertainty instead of estimating specific heights and times. Unfortunately, a few resorted to embellishment.

Despite their problems, all doctors involved in Matthew's care, from the emergency room to the medical examiner's office, agreed on the fundamental argument of the prosecution, that no disease other than acute, severe trauma could explain Matthew's illness. Madsen later told me, "I saw the kid's brain and blood. I never thought Woodward would become a cause célèbre because of it." And Mandl said "there was never any doubt" that Woodward killed Matthew, and "there still isn't." Tell any doctor about a child with a large skull fracture, a huge subdural bleed, obvious retinal hemorrhages, and a previous wrist fracture, they argue, and each will tell you the child was suddenly, violently injured.

In her book *Science on Trial*, Marcia Angell bemoans the abandonment of the scientific method in litigation involving breast implants. She finds a fundamental difference between the scientific and legal process for seeking truth. In science, one assesses data and then constructs an explanation that best fits the data, whereas in the courtroom, one decides upon a conclusion, and then presents only data that support that conclusion. Whereas Matthew's doctors examined data and presented the most likely explanation for the child's injuries when they cared for him, the defense experts assumed intentional injury never occurred and created a supporting theory. Though the defense's theory involving re-bleeding or slow progression of an old injury was highly unlikely, even unprecedented, the prosecution could never *prove* such an event never occurred. No one could.

At least one defense lawyer took the accusations of Matthew's doctors as a personal affront. In a *Wall Street Journal* commentary, Harvey Silverglate accused them of maliciously conspiring in "witchcraft." He later told me, "Once the first doctor at Children's concluded there was child abuse, others fell into line." A crusading attorney who selects only causes that interest him, Silverglate honestly believed that Woodward was railroaded; he later called the case "the single most agonizing" of his career. He based part of his skepticism of Matthew's doctors on personal experience, since his own three-week-old child had once fallen off a changing table and suffered a minor skull fracture that healed without complications. He didn't think the prosecution's misguided analogies were the product of simple courtroom naïveté, but of malignant incompetence. He said, "One of the reasons I knew the prosecution's witnesses were all wet was because they were saying that this was a kind of skull fracture that could only be inflicted from dropping a child from a two-story building onto concrete. [I] knew from personal experience that these people were complete charlatans."

Before the trial, Silverglate hired attorney Barry Scheck to assemble medical experts to argue that Matthew's death could be explained without implicating Woodward. A brilliant attorney, Scheck grasped a basic principle of courtroom science: hired experts in sufficient quantities can create the impression of legitimate scientific disagreement. He assembled a group of physicians to disagree with the Children's Hospital doctors.

On October 17, the first day of defense testimony, Barry Scheck called neuropathologist Jan Leestma, who introduced his theory that Matthew succumbed from an old, not a sudden, injury. Having concentrated on the head injury, the prosecution had not really explained Matthew's wrist fracture. Leestma hypothesized the fracture signified a previous traumatic episode that also caused a hidden brain bleed. Granted access to slides and photographs of Matthew's brain tissue after autopsy, Leestma claimed that Madsen, Matthew's neurosurgeon, had misdiagnosed Matthew's intracranial bleed as sudden when there was evidence of an extra membrane in the brain, implying a prior bleed. Leestma also asserted that he could see evidence of microscopic healing around the clot, a process that needs weeks to occur. (Later in the trial, Michael Baden, a pathologist who had previously been hired by Johnnie Cochrane for O. J. Simpson's defense, agreed with Leestma's findings.)

For purposes of the trial, Leestma appeared to have changed his mind about the significance of an extra membrane in the brain. In a neuropathology textbook published earlier, he condemned as an opportunistic defensive ploy the very testimony he gave. He wrote:

> Often there are older membranes beneath the fresh hematoma that signal prior head trauma episodes. Such older membranes are often invoked by defense attorneys to explain recent subdural hemorrhages on the basis of spontaneous re-bleeding. Such explanations do not take into consideration the brain swelling which is invariably present and the fatal outcome which [is] caused by a new episode of trauma.

During the trial, however, he contradicted himself, telling the jury that Matthew had died from exactly the type of injury he previously thought impossible. (When asked about his reversal by Martha Coakley, he said "subsequent case materials" had convinced him that his original opinion "was too narrow an interpretation.") Putting aside the speculation that an "older membrane" could ever re-bleed, three Children's Hospital pathologists and the city medical examiner who examined Matthew's brain couldn't observe any "membrane" at all, even in retrospect. To date, Leestma and Baden are the only pathologists who thought Matthew's brain had an old injury.

Leestma's testimony was important for two reasons: first, it offered a theory (however unbelievable) consistent with Matthew's wrist fracture, and second, it provided an entrée to disputing the age of Matthew's retinal hemorrhages. Previously in the trial, Lois Smith, an ophthalmologist who examined Matthew, testified for the prosecution that "the eye is witness to what's happened to the brain," and asserted that the bleeding and folding of Matthew's retinas could be caused only by severe, sudden injury. But on the second day of defense testimony, San Francisco–based neuroradiologist Alisa Gean alleged that a child could have a brain bleed that caused progressive retinal bleeding and folding over a period of weeks, a theory about retinal injury that made its debut at the trial and has never been taken seriously in any medical journal or forum. (No ophthalmologist agreed to corroborate Gean's testimony for the defense, a point used effectively by Gerard Leone in his closing argument.)

Gean also cited Madsen's operative note describing the fluid in Matthew's head as "clearish at first," implying that the fluid was old. This was an odd statement, since Madsen described a profuse amount of fresh blood in Matthew's head, and furthermore, clear fluid is expected even in sudden bleeds, since a portion of the blood can clot within minutes and leave clear yellowish fluid in its place. Though Gean rarely cares for patients directly, she said, "I have never seen an acute skull fracture without associated soft-tissue swelling." In fact, Matthew's fracture site did develop swelling by autopsy, a point that galled Ken Mandl, who had to admit Matthew initially had no external injury. "Everyone missed this simple point. It sometimes takes time to develop swelling, just like it takes time to get a bruise," he told me.

Mandl's view is supported by a widely cited 1992 study by Ann-Christine Duhaime, in which almost one-half of the cases of children with inflicted subdural bleeding had no significant evidence of external trauma. Duhaime explained that the infants' heads were hit against a "soft padded surface," like a mattress, that left no external mark of trauma. Duhaime's findings also alluded to the extreme force required to produce a retinal bleed. Of the seventy-six children with accidental injuries, only the single fatality, a passenger in a high-speed motor vehicle accident, had a retinal bleed. Of the twenty-four children with inflicted injury, nine had retinal bleeds, and three died.

Finally, the defense argued that Woodward simply wasn't strong enough to cause Matthew's injuries. For this purpose, on the third day of defense testimony Scheck called Lawrence Thibault, a biomechanics professor who studied brain injuries using animals and specially monitored dolls.

Thibault, a scientific purist who abhors any speculation, told me he thought Matthew's doctors were "full of bullshit" when they estimated the duration that Matthew was shaken or a comparable height from which he could have fallen. He thought Newberger's testimony that Matthew's eyes had "slammed back and forth in his orbits" and that his brain had "smashed back and forth within his skull" was ludicrous; he testified that "there was no slamming against the orbit."

"There is nothing more shameful than abusing a child," Thibault told me. "But as a doctor you have to be honest about what you know and don't know." Thibault legitimately corrected some misleading claims made by Matthew's doctors implying the child was solely shaken to death. But he didn't mention a key result of his studies: dolls' heads hit against an unyielding surface (such as a countertop, mattress, or floor) by adults could easily attain enough force to cause severe injuries. Based partly on these findings, the condition previously described by Caffey as "whiplash shaken baby syndrome" has been renamed "shaken baby impact syndrome."

Though Thibault correctly stated that Matthew didn't have the former condition, he should have clarified that Matthew almost certainly had the latter one. When Scheck asked if Matthew was "shaken violently, such that his neck snapped uncontrollably back and forth, be it for a period of twenty seconds or a period of about a minute," Thibault dismissed the possibility of intentional injury, and said only that Matthew "did not experience that shaking." (Defense neurosurgeons Ayub Ommaya and Ronald Uscinski supported this opinion in separate testimony.)

On October 28, closing arguments were made. Gerard Leone dramatically re-created the final moments of Matthew's life, describing how Woodward was becoming more and more upset because "Matty is still crying, he's fussy, he's cranky, and she can't stand it." He concluded, "So she grabs Matty Eappen and she shakes him because it worked before. He stopped crying. Matty Eappen stopped crying." For the defense, Andrew Good stated that Woodward was "going to go home. She's going to go back to school. Someday she'll get married and she'll be somebody's mother. And she'll be a wonderful mother." Scheck reiterated the theory that Matthew had an old injury, and added that Matthew's doctors "have been misinterpreting [data] in this case and, unfortunately, probably in other cases." Holding a CT scan of Matthew's head, Scheck said there was no swelling around Matthew's skull fracture. "This is reasonable doubt!" he exclaimed, shaking the scan. "This is the end of the case!"

The defense sensed imminent victory. Silverglate was so confident that their client would be acquitted of murder that he encouraged Woodward to ask the judge to withdraw an option for the jury to consider manslaughter, forcing a choice between murder and acquittal. The judge complied.

In a shock to Woodward's attorneys, after thirty hours of deliberation the jury convicted Woodward of second-degree murder. On Halloween, she was sentenced to life in prison. But the Woodward camp's disappointment was short-lived. Ten days later, Judge Hiller Zobel, releasing his decision via the Internet, summarily commuted the verdict to involuntary manslaughter and the penalty to time served, stating that only a slight "roughness" may have caused Matthew's death. (The following day's Boston Herald headline punned, "Saved by Zobel.") He described a version of events similar to that presented by the defense:

Had the manslaughter option been available to the jurors, they might well have selected it, not out of compromise, but because that particular verdict accorded with at least one rational view of the evidence, namely: (1) Matthew *did* indeed have a preexisting, resolving (i.e., healing) blood clot; (2) Defendant *did* handle him "roughly"; (3) the handling (although perhaps not the roughness) was intentional; (4) the force was, under the circumstances, excessive, and therefore unjustified; (5) the handling *did* cause re-bleeding; and (6) the re-bleeding caused death.

Zobel has the bearing of a patrician and the conversational style of a professor. I asked him whether he thought a courtroom was a good place to seek truth in trials involving complex medical testimony. "What is truth? The truth in a court of law," he lectured me, "is that which persuades a jury beyond a reasonable doubt." But apparently there are exceptions. For the third time in his career, he changed the decision of a jury. As in medical cases, he said, there are some times in a trial "when you can't put your finger" on what's bothersome. He wouldn't comment specifically on what bothered him in the Woodward trial, and only said vaguely, "The legal system is a human system. Things are not always perfect."

Zobel wasn't the only one who thought that the jury railroaded an innocent young woman. The *Boston Globe* praised Zobel's judicial wisdom, saying that given Matthew's preexisting bleed, the "slightest degree of mistreatment could have sufficed for a fatal injury. That rough handling would fit the definition of manslaughter. [The trial] has come to a just conclusion." The *New York Times* joined the adulation, editorializing that "Judge Zobel made use of a safety valve in Massachusetts law designed to serve justice in those rare cases when a conscientious jury produces a bad decision."

Woodward returned to her hometown of Elton, England, to a heroine's welcome, and received a crowd of well-wishers at the airport, attended parties at local pubs, and enjoyed yellow ribbons tied to trees in her honor. In contrast, Deborah Eappen, a thirty-one-year-old mother who worked part-time and arranged her schedule so that she could come home to breast-feed Matthew during the day, disposed of hate mail and was reproached by some Newton residents in *Time*. One said, "I wondered how she could leave two kids alone with an eighteen-year-old." Another commented, "An eighteen-year-old is just a child. What do you expect?"

Though Woodward had been convicted, the credence accorded to her defense during the trial infuriated many physicians, especially pediatricians. In an unprecedented decision, *Pediatrics* published a letter signed by forty-seven academic pediatricians and child abuse experts nationwide (the largest number ever permitted by the journal) that read, "The hypothesis put forward by the defense that minor trauma caused a 're-bleed' of an earlier head injury can best be characterized as inaccurate, contrary to vast clinical experience, and unsupported by any published literature. [Infants] simply do not suffer massive head injury, show no significant symptoms for days, then suddenly collapse and die." The *New England Journal of Medicine* then published an article on "nonaccidental head injury in infants" by Cindy Christian (who signed the *Pediatrics* letter) and Ann-Christine Duhaime.

The popular press largely ignored the medical community's backlash, and the search for explanations other than the most likely continued. In a trade publication naming him one of the top ten lawyers in Massachusetts a year after the trial, Harvey Silverglate suggested that Matthew may have been injured by his two-year-old brother, commenting that the defense "possibly made a mistake not bringing out that [the] older brother was imperfect. The older brother in fact was quite a wild kid."

Another sensational theory followed. Sometime in the winter of 1998, Jan Leestma, at the request of a defense lawyer, handed over pathological specimens of Matthew's brain to journalist Katie Leishman. After shopping around the tissues to several specialists nationwide, she made contact with Floyd Gilles, a neuropathologist at Children's Hospital, Los Angeles, and Marvin Nelson, chief of radiology at the same hospital. They offered yet another theory on Matthew's death, asserting he had actually been strangled, perhaps two days before his acute illness. Gilles and Nelson invoked a sort of reflexology, asserting that pressure on the neck could cause a distant artery within the head to rupture. Leishman's report aired on 60 Minutes in March 1999, and several doctors, including Bob Reece of New England Medical Center, Douglas Miller of New York University, and Eli Newberger, immediately disputed this theory.

Reviewing the many ideas about Matthew's death, one sees why even the crystal structure of DNA was described before child battery in the medical literature. Child abuse is the last possible diagnosis some people are willing to accept, occasionally for good reasons, but mostly for bad ones. As John Caffey wrote presciently decades ago, "Simple direct mechanical trauma often receives short shrift by those bent on solving the mysteries of more exotic diseases." On the wards of Children's Hospital, the residents have an aphorism for overly eager students bent on diagnosing unusual diseases instead of common problems: "When you hear hoofbeats, look for horses, not zebras." Looking for alternatives to child abuse sometimes becomes the ultimate zebra hunt.

Though painstakingly engineered over many years, public acceptance of intentional injury to children can be tenuous. How, then, can we protect children from physical battery? Predicting which infants are at risk of death is difficult. Although three million abuse and neglect reports are filed yearly, less than one in a thousand results in death. The low prevalence of fatality makes risk assessment very difficult. For example, the Department of Social Services in Salem, Massachusetts, handles about sixty calls per week regarding suspected child abuse. A social worker reviews the complaint, then interviews the family and performs a home visit, looking for indicators like social isolation, poor living conditions, previous criminal record, or previous domestic violence.

Kathleen McCarthy, the department manager, is the first to admit that many dangerous perpetrators can't be identified by these criteria. One of McCarthy's training manuals reads that abuse can sometimes "involve inflicting severe pain or torture, such as burning, starving, beating for hours, etc. [This] type of offender frequently does not have a criminal record. He is usually employed and may have a prestigious position in the community."

In his book on multiple personality disorder, *Multiple Identities and False Memories*, Nicholas Spanos describes how the witch-hunting frenzies of the seventeenth century withered once respectable people in power were accused. In many child battery cases, however, a similar dynamic allows such citizens to escape legitimate punishment. In her office overlooking the downtown where witch trials once took place, McCarthy is aware of the historical dangers of false accusations. But she has seen too many abusers escape justice and confesses that her department "simply cannot protect the children of highly intelligent sociopaths." Perhaps the lenient treatment of Woodward merely emphasizes the lesson of many sensational trials: a guilty but privileged defendant might get away with almost anything, and win public sympathy in the process.

There is, however, a more constructive viewpoint. While serious abuse certainly merits prosecution, contentious trials like that of Louise Woodward increase public distrust of the very people and institutions that help children. In truth, few cases are as obvious as that of Matthew Eappen, and, like many pediatricians, I have treated several patients with suspicious injuries but not entirely implausible stories and discharged them home to possible abusers. Bringing these cases to court would be futile, since public agency inquiries into such cases rarely reveal reasons to remove a child from the home. Ultimately, one must address the needs of these jeopardized kids.

In his 1906 short story "Sleepy-Eye," Anton Chekhov, a practicing physician, described the mental state of thirteen-year-old nanny Varka, just before she suffocated a baby:

> *"Bayu, bayushki, bayu!"* she murmurs, "Nurse will sing a song to you." But the child cries and wearies itself with crying. Varka sees again the muddy road, the men with satchels, Pelageya and father Yélim. She remembers, she recognizes them all, but in her semi-slumber she cannot understand the force which binds her, hand and foot, and crushes her, and ruins her life. She looks around her, and seeks that force that she may rid herself of it. But she cannot find it. And at last, tortured, she strains all her strength and sight; she looks upward at the winking, green spot, and as she hears the cry of the baby, she finds the enemy who is crushing her heart. The enemy is the child.

Chekhov suggests that Varka's crime results not from premeditated malice but from a defective response to stress. Today, child death review teams in Colorado and Oregon have identified specific triggers for violence, which include a child's inconsolable crying, feeding difficulty, toileting problems, and disobedience. (Woodward did tell a detective that Matthew "had been crying all day.") Rather than locating and prosecuting individual cases of abuse after they have occurred, a preemptive strategy helping caregivers learn child management skills may be better suited to dealing with potential child abuse.

At some point, every caregiver must decide whether he or she will hit a child as a disciplinary measure. Scores of psychological studies suggest that physical punishment is no more effective than time-outs, that many caregivers who hit children feel significant remorse and guilt after cooling down, and that children who are physically punished are more likely to hit their spouses and own children as adults. But like a drug, corporal punishment often results in immediate results: parents experience an acute relief of rage and a child's offending behavior is usually extinguished. It is a difficult temptation to resist, and about one-quarter of American parents hit their kids on a weekly basis. However, as with any excessive substance use, gradual tolerance may develop, requiring increasing or more frequent dosage for behavioral effect.

Perhaps by admitting that all individuals are potential abusers, strategies to prevent abuse might be identified. This effort is analogous to universal vaccination: when it's impossible to tell which children are at risk, hundreds of thousands must be inoculated against harm. The Elmira program created by David Olds in Denver uses visiting nurses and home health aides as partners with all teenage mothers for a period of six months after childbirth. The program led to an 80 percent reduction in child maltreatment in the intervention group, and a 50 percent reduction in runaways, arrests, and emergency room utilization by involved families. Though interventions like Elmira have shown positive results in multiple studies, they are present in only a handful of states.

A highlight of my second year of residency was the months attending to births at Brigham and Women's Hospital. Carrying a bright yellow tackle box full of equipment, I ran to deliveries on the obstetrics unit when a bell, indicating a high-risk birth, rang in the newborn intensive care unit. I'd arrive in the birthing room and be handed a tiny, helpless baby to resuscitate, sometimes so small that my hand was larger than its entire body.

Most times, the babies recovered in the delivery room with minimal supportive care. One of the most rewarding acts I performed was handing the infants to anxious parents, who told their baby how much they loved them, kissed them, cried tears on them, and felt such bursting joy that my own eyes misted. In contrast, one of the most depressing acts was handing the children over to mothers cursed with drug addictions, abusive relationships, or clearly unwanted and resented pregnancies.

Sunil Eappen, whose specialty is obstetrical anesthesia, was often present attending to the mother's anesthesia for cesarean sections. Sometimes I watched his face, wondering what he was thinking, witnessing over and over the drama of childbirth. I couldn't bring myself ever to ask him. Perhaps he felt the same thing I did: a searing desire to convince at-risk families what a delicate vessel a child is, so in need of nurturing, and so fragile.

~ 5 ~

Brain

ON THE ACCEPTANCE AND TAMING OF DANGER

In the Huancayo highlands of northern Peru, my friend David Lauer and I wrestled a pig to the ground for the purpose of preventing seizures in children. It was a wonderful way to pass a brisk spring morning. After surveying an open field market, we bought alpaca blankets and received a lesson on lamb slaughtering from a leathery old-timer. We drank warm mugs of *café con leche* and we got to work. Because he wasn't feeling well, David took two tablets of ibuprofen.

That morning his fever had hit 104 degrees Fahrenheit. He seemed particularly unlucky. The week before he had narrowly escaped death when Shining Path terrorists bombed a bungalow near our quarters outside Lima. Now he had come down with typhoid. This followed a recent attack of schistosomiasis in Malawi. Bizarre health problems seemed to assault David everywhere; when we went scuba diving near Venezuela a few years later, a sea wasp stung his wrist and caused the skin to slough off. But David was unflappable; he shrugged off his ailments as the price of living an interesting life.

Shepherds and pig farmers brought their livestock for sale to the field, and we were particularly interested in one pig. David held down the large animal while I forcibly inserted a wooden dowel into its mouth. *Say ahh*, I thought. The pig had a peculiar pattern of nodules under the tongue. The animal was perfect for our purpose, so we paid the weathered owner seventy soles and became the proud owners of a Huancayo hog. Now we only needed four more like it.

A worm called *Taenia solium* had caused the lesions on the pig's tongue. Most highlanders knew about this parasite. That's why they sold these pigs cheaply; no one else wanted them. Unselective about their diet, pigs acquire the infection by eating human feces contaminated by *Taenia* eggs. The acid in the pig's stomach dissolves the egg's shell and liberates an embryo, which burrows through the stomach wall to enter the pig's bloodstream. Because a pig may eat thousands of microscopic eggs at once, the parasite embryos disperse like confetti, hitching rides from the circulation to the pig's tongue, muscles, liver, and other organs. Over time these settlers develop into larvae called cysticerci, which can form the telltale lesions on pigs' tongues. This condition is called cysticercosis.

But the only place that the cysticerci lay eggs is inside a human's gut. When humans eat infected pork that has been undercooked, the cysticerci pass alive into the intestines and grow as long as twelve feet. The parasite's relatively small head attaches to the gut wall, and the balance of the body dangles freely through the small intestine like the tail of a kite. The worm looks like a link of sausages, and periodically one of the links breaks off the end and passes in the person's stool. This link or "proglottid" contains forty

thousand to fifty thousand *Taenia* eggs. In areas without plumbing—such as Huancayo—pigs eat infected human excrement left in
open fields, acquire cysticercosis, are consumed by humans, and
thus continue the cycle.

Finding other infected pigs at the market wasn't difficult. When
word spread that two gringos were buying pigs with tongue lesions,
we were fairly mobbed by sellers. Four wrestling bouts later, David
and I had filled our quota. Now came the hard part. The return trip
to Lima would last five hours, and all we had for transport was an
old Chevy Impala. One by one, David and I subdued the pigs and
forced a white sedative into their snouts. Then we loaded the unconscious pigs into the trunk and closed it. I nursed a bruise on my face.
While leaving, I spied an unexpected entertainment: a man had a
foosball table in the center of the sheep slaughtering area. David and I
paid a sol to introduce our companions Valerie and Paola to the
game, and we happily spun small plastic soccer figures in the midst
of the gore.

Though one of the pigs died in the trunk on the return trip, the
rest were fine. At the veterinary clinic we dropped them off with
Lallo and Marcos, who were running experiments using a drug
called oxfendazole, which might have prevented the problem I saw
a few years later.

The life cycle of *Taenia solium* became particularly important to me
in the emergency room one day in Boston. An ambulance pulled up
and the paramedics brought in a stretcher on which a five-year-old
boy thrashed his arms and legs uncontrollably. His head was
twisted to the right, and he didn't respond when we touched him or
called to him. "He was at school and started doing this at recess
about ten minutes ago," the paramedic reported. The child was having a seizure.

The brain is a network of cells called neurons, which interconnect in nearly unfathomable fashion to control our actions and synthesize consciousness. In the words of economist Thomas Schelling, a free society is "an ecology of micromotives," where independent people with various motivations interact in many environments. Similarly the brain is like a society where neurons exchange information in trillions of isolated transactions. In large economies, Schelling thought that a few people—in the right place at the right time—could unexpectedly conspire to form coalitions, monopolies, and, rarely, dictatorships. Likewise, a seizure is a totalitarian transformation of the brain—a system of free transactions gone wrong—where large areas of the brain are forced into a state of exaggerated synchronization by a few nerves gone bad.

About one in five Americans has such an event—a seizure—at some time, and epilepsy, or recurrent seizures, is the second most common brain disorder, surpassed only by stroke. Seizures have various manifestations. Most of the time, the seizure is "partial" and occurs in a localized area of the brain. An individual may have involuntary jerking of an arm or leg. Sometimes people hear buzzing noises, see flashes of light, have déjà vu, or feel the abdominal sensation of going down a roller coaster. Two thousand years ago, Hippocrates described a man who felt a breeze (the Greek for breeze is *aura*) over his arm. This patient then developed loss of consciousness. In this man the localized area of seizure likely kindled the brain's awareness center and caused altered consciousness, resulting in a "complex-partial" seizure. Patients with complex-partial seizures frequently feel warning sensations such as breezes and funny smells or tastes (now generically referred to as auras) before losing consciousness. Though unaware of their actions, a person may still perform complex, stereotyped behaviors called automatisms. Among other types, their seizures may be cursive (characterized by frantic running) or gelastic (characterized by uncontrollable laughing). In Michael Crichton's bestseller *The Terminal Man*, the fictional protagonist suffers from complex-partial seizures characterized by paroxysms of homicidal rage, a plausible scenario.

Other times, a seizure is not partial but "generalized," meaning that the conflagration involves the entire brain. The individual loses consciousness, and the whole body may convulse in a coordinated manner. Known alternately as *grand mal* or tonic-clonic convulsions, these seizures are dramatic. Occasionally no limb movements are seen, and these generalized seizures are known as "absence" or *petit mal* seizures. Other than these, there are about two dozen other seizure disorders; perhaps the most frightening to parents is the rare Landau-Kleffner syndrome. A healthy child between the ages of three and eight suddenly becomes mute, sometimes in a matter of days. Often these children are misdiagnosed as autistic or mentally retarded, but actually they suffer from a form of epilepsy.

The child in the emergency room, Fernando Garcia, was having a generalized tonic-clonic seizure. We brought him into the trauma bay, hooked him up to monitors, took his temperature, and measured the oxygen levels in his blood. His vitals signs were stable, implying that his heart and lungs were functioning well despite the seizure. Fernando didn't have a fever, which ruled out a simple febrile seizure. These occur in children six months to five years old, are accompanied by fever (which is thought to cause the seizure), are always generalized, and usually require no treatment.

We had to act quickly because seizures that go on for too long— over thirty to forty-five minutes—can cause permanent brain injury. When nerves fire repetitively for a long time, too much neurotransmitter, the chemical that nerves release to communicate with one another, accumulates in the brain. This excess can kill nerves.

In 1987, a Canadian outbreak of prolonged seizures followed the consumption of cultivated mussels from Prince Edward Island. Several patients died. The problem was traced to the mussels' contamination by marine vegetation that produced domoic acid, a potent neurotransmitter. Fernando, instead of eating a neurotransmitter, was releasing too much of his own domoic acid by having a prolonged seizure. This was just as dangerous, since 20 percent of people who have a prolonged seizure die. The Canadian episode emphasized the role of excess neurotransmitters in causing brain damage, and by implication the need to stop their release in Fernando's brain.

"Can I have lorazepam, three milligrams please?" I asked the nurse, who drew the medication into a slender syringe and injected it into Fernando's IV. Closely related to the tranquilizer Valium (which until recently was the most prescribed medication in the country), lorazepam promotes sleep. In four out of five people, it works in a few minutes.

I checked my watch. Fernando's limbs continued to thrash. He had an unpleasant odor, having moved his bowels involuntarily. It is exceedingly uncomfortable to watch a child seize; one's instinct is to do something, anything. But we had to wait five minutes to see if the lorazepam had any effect. It didn't. We gave a second dose and waited another five minutes, but Fernando kept on seizing.

"Could we please get phenytoin, six hundred milligrams intravenous please?" I asked the nurse. Phenytoin is a type of barbiturate or sedative developed after 1912, when A. Hauptman noted that psychiatric patients sedated with barbiturates had fewer seizures. The pharmaceutical company Parke-Davis in 1953 then created nineteen different forms of barbiturates and found, in a stroke of luck, that the very first one that was tested, phenytoin, stopped seizures provoked by electric shocks to animals' brains. (The story of valproic acid, another key antiepileptic drug, is even more remarkable. When Berthier Laboratories of France found that every single medication they tested seemed to stop seizures, an astute scientist figured out that the solvent they used for the testing—valproic acid—and not the medications made by the company was the active substance.)

The phenytoin was infused over a few minutes, and Fernando's jerking slowed and finally stopped. I rubbed Fernando's chest and spoke loudly into his ear, but he still didn't respond. That was probably all right, as people just recovering from seizures remain unresponsive for several minutes. I was pleased that the phenytoin worked, since our only other option to stop the seizure was to purposely put Fernando into a coma with extremely high doses of barbiturates.

Fernando's mother, a Mexican immigrant, arrived from work where she was a seamstress. I brought two chairs to Fernando's bedside and we reviewed what happened. Neither her English nor my Spanish were passable. An interpreter was paged and meanwhile Fernando woke up, back to his usual self. He didn't remember the seizure at all. When the interpreter arrived, Fernando's mother held her son on her lap tightly and asked the question so many parents ask when their children fall ill: "Why did this happen?"

There were many reasons, I explained. The most common reason to have a seizure was fever, since almost one in twenty children under the age of five with a high fever will seize. However, Fernando didn't have a fever. The absence of fever also made meningitis, or an infection of the brain's lining, extremely unlikely. That meant that Fernando was one of about thirty thousand children a year who have an "afebrile" seizure.

In young children, many triggers could cause one. I reviewed the causes. Some newborn infants fed excessive plain water can dilute the sodium content of their blood, causing severe seizures. (This is one reason babies should drink only breast milk or formula until four months of age.) Rarely, diabetics who receive too much insulin, malnourished children who have rickets, or neglected children who somehow ingest cocaine develop seizures. However, Fernando's blood and urine tests ruled out these conditions. Another possibility was that the boy had a "twitchy" region in the brain, which can be identified by a brain wave study, or electroencephalogram (EEG).

Offhand, I asked if Fernando played many video games or watched a lot of cartoons. On December 16, 1997, an episode of the cartoon show *Pokémon* aired in Japan, and in many prefectures almost 70 percent of elementary school students watched. About twenty minutes into the program, the character Pikachu used his electric powers to stop a "virus bomb," depicted by a series of flashing lights. Within forty minutes, over six hundred children were taken to hospitals for reported seizures, caused by so-called photo-sensitivity epilepsy or PSE. (The outbreak was also a classic example of group hysteria; later thousands of Japanese children were taken to hospitals for all kinds of symptoms attributed to the episode.) This wasn't the first episode of television-induced PSE; following an outbreak of seizures after a noodle commercial in 1993, British television began restricting flashes in commercials to three per second. But Fernando had no history of such an exposure.

Finally—and I hesitated to say this to Fernando's mother—a tumor within Fernando's head could cause a seizure. While an MRI scan is the best way to look for these, we could get a CT scan immediately to rule out any obvious problems. We often needed to wait several days to schedule an MRI, so a CT scan was the fastest strategy now. The bottom line, though, was that most children who develop seizures have no identifiable cause; all blood tests, urine tests, EEGs, and brain scans are normal. When this happens, children generally go home with no treatment and are medicated only if seizures recur.

The nurse wheeled Fernando to the CT scanner, and within ten minutes I received an urgent page from the radiologist. "You have to come see this," he said. I walked to the radiology suite and we looked at the images. There were two apricot-sized cysts on the right side of Fernando's brain. One of the cysts had small flecks of calcium in it. The radiologist called the chief of the department, who reviewed the films and stroked his forehead. "Well," he concluded, "it seems the child has cysticercosis of the brain."

We wondered how Fernando had gotten this infection. Scientists have known that pork consumption is related to cysticercosis; the disease is almost unknown in many Muslim countries, where the Koran forbids pork consumption. But in 1990, a small epidemic of brain cysticercosis occurred in an Orthodox Jewish community in New York, which was puzzling. Judaism, like Islam, forbids pork consumption. How had these people acquired the illness? An investigation by the U.S. Centers for Disease Control revealed that each affected person employed illegal Latin American immigrants for domestic assistance, and these workers had intestinal *Taenia solium* larvae that laid eggs, which passed in the stool. Because the workers practiced poor hand washing, their hands were contaminated with these eggs, which found their way into their employers' foods.

It is important to point out that the domestic workers did *not* have cysticercosis, or worms throughout their bodies, as did the infected pigs they had eaten in their homeland. Rather, they had only intestinal colonization with the worms that laid eggs. To get cysticercosis in the brain, a person must eat not a larva (as from an infected animal) but an egg (from the stool of a human) whose covering is dissolved in the stomach, allowing an embryo to burrow through the stomach, enter the bloodstream, and reach the brain. Fernando had thus eaten an egg at some point, which came from a household contact that had a worm in the intestine. This happened all the time; studies have shown that almost half of people with epilepsy in Latin American countries have neurocysticercosis.

I walked back to the emergency room and broke the news to Fernando's mother. She was familiar with the illness; her brother had suffered from *nerviosimo* (a folk term for a seizure or a nerve problem) and had been treated unsuccessfully by a folk healer called a *cuarandero* with a multitude of remedies. I explained the cause of Fernando's seizures and admitted him to the ward for observation. I called the neurologist, who recommended continued phenytoin to prevent further seizures. Then I called the infectious disease specialist for advice on any helpful antibiotics.

Like many pediatricians, I often ask for assistance with complicated cases. While information technology places vast amounts of information at a clinician's disposal (I currently subscribe to several Internet reference services that contain gigabyte upon gigabyte of literature), there is no substitute for talking directly with an experienced specialist. For a single child, a pediatrician may consult eight or more specialists, like cardiologists, pulmonologists, gastroenterologists, nephrologists, and so on. Each specialist contributes an enriched analysis of a particular organ, and it is the pediatrician's job to put it together.

The infectious disease expert explained that the role of antibiotics in neurocysticercosis was controversial; no one knew if they helped. However, she concluded that Fernando should try an antibiotic called praziquantel. This would kill the worms in his brain, even though no one knew if the cysts would then disappear or whether the worms' remains would stay in Fernando's brain all his life. This might not even make his seizures better. Fernando would live his life with the constant danger of recurrent seizures, since no one knew if his brain would heal.

However, perhaps other children could be protected from acquiring Fernando's illness in the first place. Public health programs are based on prevention. The first modern public health intervention took place in 1854 when the British queen's physician, John Snow, deduced that a single sewage-contaminated well was responsible for a deadly cholera outbreak. As the story goes, he removed the handle from the well's pump and immediately halted the epidemic. Almost one hundred fifty years later David Lauer and I also assisted in the prevention of infection from poor sewage disposal, this time by wrestling pigs.

To understand why control of *Taenia solium* is difficult, it's useful to review a disease of the nervous system that is more easily eradicated: polio. An extraordinary effort is under way to erase polio globally; in fact, the last naturally occurring case in the entire

Western Hemisphere occurred in Peru in 1991. Gone are the days when gymnasium-sized rooms at Children's Hospital were filled with children in "iron lungs," or artificial respirator devices. (Once when I was lost in the basement of the hospital, I ran across an old, rusted iron lung in an abandoned room.) This public health success occurred for three reasons. First, an effective, oral vaccine was available; second, there was no animal "reservoir" of virus that could secretly harbor the infection; and finally, there was a concerted political and public health campaign directed against polio. In the case of cysticercosis, none of these features are present. Hence we struck the disease at its most accessible point, in pigs.

People who eat *Taenia solium* eggs (from fecal-oral contact with other humans) get the worms in their brains and other areas, but aren't contagious. Only people who eat infected pork acquire the worm in their intestines and pass eggs in their stools. Thus, controlling the parasite in pigs can stop the disease's transmission.

The pigs that David and I brought back from Huancayo were treated with an experimental antiparasitic agent called oxfendazole. The researchers with whom we worked discovered that a single dose of the drug completely killed all worms within the pig. Any pig with the parasite can be treated with oxfendazole, and later be eaten safely. This approach—targeting an animal vector for intervention, instead of people—has also been used to control rabies (by immunizing dogs), malaria (by killing mosquitoes), and other illnesses. In certain Peruvian areas of endemic infection, newborn "sentinel" pigs are placed in strategic areas. After a year, researchers examine them to see if they have acquired cysticercocis. By focusing on areas where a large number of pigs become newly infected, health authorities can determine what areas have the highest levels of sewage contamination and target greater efforts to treat pigs with oxfendazole or aggressively improve sanitation.

Although these efforts are still in their infancy, they're a start to protect children like Fernando from a possible lifetime of epilepsy.

~~~

While Fernando Garcia had a problem with the *function* of the brain, nine-year-old Laurie Manygoats had a problem with the *structure* of the brain. I met her shortly after moving to Gallup, New Mexico, to work with Navajo children in the U.S. Indian Health Service. The largest remaining tribe in the United States, the Navajo claim 130,000 members scattered across a reservation larger than West Virginia. The Navajo refer to themselves as the Diné, which can be translated as "earth people." I lived just down the road from the hospital on Nizhoni Boulevard, a street named after the Navajo word for "walking in beauty." Every action and every component of the world has a spiritual meaning to a traditional Navajo; to "walk in beauty" is to experience the full grace of existence.

Despite the spiritual richness of Navajo culture, many problems exist on the reservation. The breathtaking local scenery hides significant environmental contamination. In the 1970s at Church Rock, a town northeast of Gallup, a poorly built dam at the United Nuclear Corporation failed, sending 95 million gallons of contaminated water and 1,100 tons of radioactive mud into town. The public water is still contaminated with traces of uranium. Unemployment on the reservation fluctuates between one-third and one-half of the entire population. Ten years ago, the television newsmagazine *20/20* dubbed Gallup "Drunk Town, U.S.A." Though Gallup is a border town with only 20,000 permanent residents, its population swells to several times this number on weekends. Alcohol abuse is rampant; in the 1980s, almost 34,000 people yearly were taken to the local drunk tank (perhaps the largest single jail cell in the United States) for detoxification. On my very first day as the on-call pediatrician, I presided over the unsuccessful resuscitation of a two-year-old whose spinal cord was sheared in an alcohol-related auto accident, riding without a car seat. What was I seeking in a place like this? In his novel *The Quincunx*, Charles Palliser writes, "The rose is safe within the thorns." Perhaps that's why I was drawn to Navajo country: despite its veneer of danger, there was a promise of beauty.

Laurie first came to the pediatric clinic with her mother because of a swelling in her neck. After doing blood tests and speaking with an endocrinologist, I concluded that Laurie had a viral infection of her thyroid gland, which should have improved spontaneously. But when Laurie returned after six weeks, her thyroid wasn't any smaller. This was puzzling, and I was reminded of an old medical aphorism particularly relevant in today's age of high technology: when in doubt, talk to the patient.

So I set aside an hour and we just talked. Laurie lived in a place called Twin Lakes, about forty miles into the reservation. Her family was traditional; they lived in an earthen octagonal dwelling called a hogan, hauled water from a nearby well, and had no electricity or telephone service. A perky girl, Laurie told me about herding sheep (an activity she loved) and her favorite food, mutton stew. She didn't like the yellow dog that chased her home every day from the school bus stop. Also, she didn't like it when the kids at school called her "Bigfoot." Her mother explained that Laurie was much taller than the other girls in her class.

Hearing this, I plotted Laurie's height and weight on a growth chart and noticed the nine-year-old was the average size of a fifteen-year-old. Compared to her growth as an infant (I requested records from a previous pediatrician), Laurie's size reflected an explosive increase in growth beginning at the age of five years. A child's growth is normally so consistent that a two-year-old is exactly half her adult height and grows with unerring predictability; a significant deviation in growth velocity causes concern.

A child's growth depends largely on a pea-sized part of the brain called the pituitary gland. If the head were a sphere, the gland would sit in its center, behind the bridge of the nose. A thin stalk of nerves connects the pituitary to another part of the brain called the hypothalamus. The center of emotion, the hypothalamus bridges the animal spinal cord (which essentially controls reflexes and has no cognitive function) to the uniquely human cerebral cortex (which is the repository of thought). The cerebral cortex looks like a large cauliflower sprouting from the thick stem of the hypothalamus, which in turn connects to the long root of the brain stem.

Composed of 100 to 200 billion nerves, the brain has a functional organization first outlined by Wilder Penfield in a remarkable series of experiments in the 1950s. A neurosurgeon interested in epilepsy, Penfield was the first to realize that the brain itself has no pain fibers and thus he used only local anesthesia on patients undergoing brain surgery. By jolting areas of the brain with a small electric current and asking patients what they felt, Penfield tried to reproduce the auras that preceded a seizure. If a patient felt the aura with stimulation in a particular place, Penfield destroyed that tiny part of brain. In many patients, this maneuver cured epilepsy. What was astonishing was what Penfield found as a by-product of these surgeries. When he stimulated a specific part of the cerebral cortex, a patient remembered a particular song, taste, or smell from their childhood. He discovered that memories have a physical location. Furthermore, he mapped areas of the brain to the parts of the body they control. A representation called the homunculus, or miniature human being, often portrays this map. This cartoon has body parts drawn proportionately to how much brain space they occupy. For example, the figure's lips, fingers, and genitals with their high number of nerve endings are much larger than its limbs.

Since Penfield, the function of the brain has been mapped in exquisite detail; today an abnormality of a person's reflexes, cognition, memory, or motor function can be traced to a specific region of malfunction in the brain.

Suspecting that Laurie's sudden growth implied a neurological problem, I first tested her reflexes by tapping on each of her joints.

They weren't too brisk (as in excess thyroid hormone production) or too sluggish (as in vitamin B_{12} deficiency). This meant that her spinal cord and nerves outside the brain were likely normal.

I had Laurie close her eyes and stand, and gently pushed her to the side. She maintained her balance well. After opening her eyes, Laurie flipped her hands repeatedly, like pancakes turned rapidly back and forth. These tests demonstrated that her cerebellum, a golf ball–sized protrusion off the rear of the brain stem, controlled her coordination well. After additional tests of her limb movements, short-term memory, speech, and additional reflexes, I was satisfied that most of her brain—at least by physical exam—was normal.

The final part of the exam was the eyes. The eyes' relation to the brain is so complex that an entire medical subspecialty, neuro-ophthalmology, is devoted to the subject. Laurie removed her glasses and sat on the exam table. I took an ophthalmoscope and flashed the bright light at her pupils. The lenses of her eyes focused the light onto her retina, where the light energy was converted to an electrical impulse by remarkable cells called photoreceptors or, more popularly, rods and cones. (Some researchers believe that even a *single* photon—the small, massless particle that makes up light—can be sensed by a photoreceptor.) The impulse traveled through the optic nerve, crossed to the opposite side of the brain at the optic chiasm, and entered the midbrain, just behind the hypo-thalamus. There, at an area called the Edinger-Westphal nucleus, the message was processed and an order was issued. The order was telegraphed back to a sphincter muscle in the eye. Seeing Laurie's pupil constrict, I knew that this entire neural pathway was intact. Laurie then focused on a small hand puppet, which I moved closer and closer until reaching the bridge of her nose. Her eyes were crossed, and also constricted just as when I had shined a bright light on them. This was another normal reflex. In 1869, Douglas Argyll Robertson noticed that some patients with syphilis in the brain had an abnormal reaction to bright light but normal constriction with fixation on a near object. Today, we know this reflects a problem in the midbrain. But Laurie's midbrain seemed fine.

I was particularly interested in Laurie's midbrain because it houses the hypothalamus, on which the pituitary gland hangs. That was where Laurie's problem must lie. But so far nothing seemed amiss. So why was she so tall, and how was this related to her neck mass?

It must have something to do with growth hormone, which is made by the pituitary gland. Too much growth hormone could explain both her height and the swelling of her thyroid. In an average girl, the pituitary remains in hibernation until about eight to nine years of age. At that time, the hypothalamus kick starts puberty by activating the pituitary gland. (A widely cited study by Marcia Herman-Giddens found that this is happening significantly earlier today, prompting debate on the reason for earlier puberty. Possible causes include better nutrition, environmental contamination with estrogens, and obesity, to name a few.) In addition to other hormones, the pituitary secretes increasing amounts of growth hormone, and the child experiences a growth spurt. But Laurie had no associated signs of puberty such as breast buds or pubic hair. Therefore, something other than puberty was driving her pituitary's production of growth hormone.

I looked again at Laurie. She had a somewhat broad nose and coarse facial features. Her fingers were thick. These were classic features of gigantism, or acromegaly. Several famous people have had this condition, including the horror movie actor Rondo Hatton, wrestler Andre "The Giant" Rousimoff, and actor Carel Struycken, who played Lurch in *The Addams Family* movie. Ben-Gurion University neurologist Vladimir Berginer believes that the biblical giant Goliath also had acromegaly, a condition that (for reasons I'll clarify) may have prevented him from seeing David's stone flying at his generous skull.

I had examined Laurie so painstakingly because I was convinced she had a large brain tumor, likely in the pituitary gland or in the hypothalamus, which would result in an abnormal eye exam or other discernible physical problems. Such a tumor would cause large amounts of growth hormone to be released, causing Laurie's acromegaly and also her excessive thyroid growth. Given her normal exam, the only way to be sure now was to obtain an MRI of her brain, which would take a week.

After we sat down with Laurie's mother, I outlined the results of Laurie's exam, and gradually came around to her likely diagnosis. It took about fifteen minutes until I said, "I think, and I'm not absolutely sure until we can see an MRI, that Laurie has a problem in her brain that's causing her to grow too fast. This problem is probably a tumor."

Laurie began to cry, and her mother looked ahead with a frown. I've given bad news or seen bad news broken often enough to expect a variety of reactions from patients. As the instrument of bad news, I often remember the same words that J. Robert Oppenheimer did upon seeing the detonation of the world's first atomic weapon, taken from the Hindu scripture *Bhagavad-Gita* when the deity Krishna assumes his most ominous incarnation: "I am become Death, the destroyer of worlds." This metaphor is mutual; patients told about cancers or other terrible conditions refer to the day the "bomb dropped."

"Is that," Laurie said between sobs, "why I've been having such bad headaches?" She hadn't mentioned this before. I nodded silently. "I thought," she continued, "that the skin-walkers were trying to get me."

In a stream of consciousness, Laurie kept talking: "At night they come to my room, and they don't have eyes and they get in through the cracks in the window and they say they're going to kill me and my mother even tried a ceremony to keep them away and it didn't work. And so I always wear my cross at night and it still doesn't help. And I asked my grandmother to come down from heaven and last night she did and I saw an angel who said I'll be all right and I went to sleep but I'm still so scared."

There was more. Still crying, she said, "Sometimes I'm sitting in class and they come to me and no one else sees them and they talk to me and tell me they're going to kill me and take my eyes. Then I see a flash of light and I feel cold and they're gone. So I pray hard and pray and they sometimes get scared and the skinny-walkers stay away and then I pretend the angel is back and looking over me and then I'm happy but then at night the skin-walkers come back and I'm still scared." Laurie took a tissue to dab her eyes and her mother said, "Why didn't you tell me all of this, Laurie?"

Laurie had been hoarding religious artifacts such as crosses and prayer beads for several weeks, explained her mother. Her daughter was afraid of sleeping alone, which was new for her. I thought of Haley Joel Osment's character from *The Sixth Sense*, who was also tormented by visions of skin-walkers, or undead spirits. Like him, she had developed her own rituals to protect herself, using whatever spiritual artifacts she could collect. Laurie had to cope with extraordinary fear. I tried to reassure her that the spirits she saw were not real; they were illusions probably related to her brain tumor. But I don't think this explanation helped her very much.

We scheduled the MRI and performed some blood tests. When Laurie returned with her mother one week later, we reviewed the results. Her MRI showed a plum-sized tumor that obscured the pituitary gland and hypothalamus. The tumor also encased the optic nerve, which slightly harmed Laurie's ability to see. When we performed a computerized test of Laurie's visual fields that day, we found that she had some mild tunnel vision, a typical finding in pituitary tumors. (This is the reason Goliath may not have been able to see the projectile that hit him.) Earlier I had also sent the MRI to a neurosurgeon in Albuquerque, and his opinion was discouraging—the tumor was too large to be operable. A surgery would likely leave

Laurie blind and perhaps even kill her. In addition, Laurie's blood tests showed that the tumor was making two types of pituitary hormones, growth hormone (which caused acromegaly) and another called prolactin. This was highly unusual, and a search of Medline showed only a handful of such cases in children.

Thankfully, Laurie had an option other than surgery. There are substances known that kill nerves right near Laurie's tumor. For example, in the 1980s, a careless drug dealer in California caused an outbreak of Parkinson's disease among otherwise healthy addicts by contaminating a batch of designer drugs with a substance called MPTP, which destroys nerves in the midbrain. In Laurie's case, though, giving MPTP would be like amputating a leg to cure an ingrown toenail. There was a more elegant approach. After all, we didn't really want to destroy the midbrain; we just wanted to change the signals it sent to the pituitary.

The midbrain—in particular, the hypothalamus—controls the pituitary gland. When the hypothalamus lacks a chemical called dopamine, the pituitary gland activates and secretes prolactin and growth hormone, which Laurie had in excess quantities. But when the hypothalamus is bathed in dopamine, the pituitary gland becomes quiescent and stops releasing these hormones. Laurie might be helped if we could get extra dopamine into her midbrain and stop her pituitary gland's profligate dumping of hormones.

In recent years, drugs that do exactly this were discovered. I called an endocrinologist, who recommended initiating a dopamine-like medication called cabergoline approved for use in pituitary tumors. It's a small pill that Laurie would take twice a week. Somewhat cynically, I wondered if such a simple treatment could control a brain tumor. We'd see soon enough.

Laurie came to see me weekly for the next month, and she had no significant side effects from the medication. Though the nocturnal hallucinations still occurred, they were a little less frightening to her. Laurie's mother gave me an update on the home front. She had arranged weekly healing ceremonies with a medicine man, who conducted them in sweat lodges with Navajo elders. At night, Laurie wore protective bracelets with religious inscriptions. Like many parents with sick children, Laurie's mother pulled out all spiritual stops; she requested prayers at the local Baptist church in addition to the Navajo ceremonies. I also was told that Laurie's schoolteacher requested that no child use epithets like "Bigfoot" and held a special meeting with her students to explain Laurie's illness.

After one month of cabergoline treatment, Laurie had another MRI and series of blood tests. While waiting for the films to be brought from radiology, Laurie and I talked about her favorite series of books, about the boy wizard Harry Potter. She particularly remembered a scene where Harry Potter's class learns to fight magical creatures called *boggarts*, shape-shifters that scare children by assuming the form of what they dread most. A young wizard defeats a boggart by mentally visualizing something humorous and exclaiming, *"Riddikulus!"* Laurie was trying this at night with her tormentors; when the eyeless ghouls came, she pictured them in funny ballet costumes and yelled the charm, and they sometimes vanished.

When the films arrived, I hung them on a light-box next to the previous ones from the month earlier. Laurie and her mother stood next to me and we eagerly looked at them. The results were astounding. The tumor had—in the span of only one month— shrunk in volume by almost 50 percent. Later the blood tests returned to show that her levels of pituitary hormones had decreased by a proportional amount. I was so excited I gave Laurie and her mother bear hugs and called the endocrinologist who recommended the treatment to share the news. She explained that once deprived of stimulation from the hypothalamus, the pituitary tumor begins to die of neglect. This was common in tumors that were dependent on hormone or neurotransmitter secretion (for example, like certain types of breast and prostate cancer); the tumor can't survive without nurturing. Cabergoline somehow cut the tumor's supply lines in Laurie's brain.

After further discussion with a neurosurgeon and the endocrinologist, I elected to continue the cabergoline, and a third MRI after another month of therapy showed continued tumor shrinkage. Laurie's headaches and hallucinations were markedly better. The tumor was the size of a grape instead of a plum, and the neurosurgeon thought he might be able to remove it soon. Laurie would have to live with the tumor in her head a little longer, but it was now a waning danger.

In a recent visit, Laurie asked me if I had a Navajo dream-catcher for my son, who was due in a few weeks. I didn't. A dream-catcher is a circle of metal with a spiderweb pattern of thread stretched over it. It is placed at the head of a baby's crib, where it is said to intercept nightmares and allow the passage of only happy dreams. "Maybe I'll make him a dream-catcher," she said, smiling. "I think everybody needs one."

Laurie's problem was highly unusual. School failure, on the other hand, is a common problem that affects many children.

Damien Jones was an eleven-year-old boy called "difficult" by his fifth-grade teacher. He didn't get along well with his peers, and did poorly in group activities. He rarely sat still at his desk, and frequently interrupted his teacher with outbursts in the middle of a lesson. Recently, he had raised his hand and waved it back and forth with such insistent force that he fell out of his chair. Damien's desk was filled with a disorganized array of worksheets, and though he owned a binder, it remained empty. "Damien possesses obvious intelligence, but has serious organizational and attention problems," wrote his teacher on his last report card. He was failing several subjects. An average-sized boy with sandy brown hair, Damien was brought by his mother to the developmental evaluation center at Children's Hospital after a particularly bad quarter at school.

These evaluations frequently made me feel like a law enforcement officer interrogating a suspect. While another pediatric resident named Tamika Joseph asked questions and played testing "games" with Damien, a developmental specialist and I watched him through a one-way mirror from a concealed room. A hidden speaker system transmitted sound to us. I sipped a cup of black coffee and jotted notes. Just the facts, I thought.

After several weeks of watching these evaluations, I had developed a healthy suspicion of the motives of some parents. I occasionally thought they wanted to secure (regardless of the test results) a label of a learning disability for their child, who could then obtain additional services at school. I suppose this was to be expected; pediatricians acted as the gatekeepers to special education services such as individualized tutorials, counseling, untimed tests, and other help sought by some parents for their children.

Special education services are mandated for all eligible children by a series of federal and state laws. In 1973, Congress passed the Rehabilitation Act, which includes Section 504, a law guaranteeing special educational services to children deemed functionally "handicapped," a term that includes any type of learning disability. This right to education was enhanced in 1975 when Congress passed what is today called the Individuals with Disabilities Education Act, or IDEA, which extended special education services to all children, including those with major disabilities such as blindness. To better define what specific guarantees were made to disabled children, the Supreme Court in 1982 ruled in *Board of Education v. Rowley* that an "appropriate" educational program for a disabled child implies one that offers "educational benefit." This is typically defined (for those with mild disabilities) as ensuring that a child makes passing grades in an age-appropriate classroom. The exact definition of "educational benefit," however, is left to the states.

In most states today, a parent, teacher, or principal can initiate a diagnostic evaluation for a child simply by writing a letter containing the words, "I am writing to make a referral for assessment for special education services." Within a defined period of time (typically a few weeks), a school district must perform a comprehensive battery of psychological and learning tests to decide whether or not a disability exists. If parents disagree with a school's initial diagnosis, or if the school psychologists need further diagnostic assistance, a child is guaranteed another evaluation by a third party at the school district's expense. (That's where our hospital came in. Children were generally brought to us for a second opinion.) If a disability is identified by the school district or the third-party evaluation, the school district has about two months to develop an Individualized Education Plan, or IEP. The actual instrument of a child's special education, an IEP prescribes in detail the child's services, such as speech therapy, untimed tests, counseling, or other interventions to ensure that the child derives "educational benefit" from school in the "least restrictive environment."

Two months ago, Damien's school district diagnosed him with a conduct disorder, meaning that he had discipline problems. His IEP included visits with the school counselor twice a week. Unsatisfied with her son's progress with the counselor, Damien's mother requested a second opinion from us.

Behind the one-way mirror, I watched Damien work through a series of written problems. His eyes were intense and brown, and his well-formed mouth was briefly pursed in concentration. I glanced at his intake form and noted that his height and weight were normal. Based on a child's appearance, we periodically identify a child with a previously missed genetic problem, usually involving the sex chromosomes of which girls normally have two X types (XX) and boys have one X and one Y type (XY). However, sometimes girls have only a single X chromosome (XO), a condition called Turner's syndrome. These girls have abnormally shaped necks, short stature, delayed puberty, and usually mild mental retardation. A boy with a thin face, poor school performance, and aggressive tendencies might have an extra Y chromosome (XYY) and have Klinfelter's syndrome. Nongenetic problems might also be possible; for example, widely spaced eyes, thin lips, and school failure could indicate fetal alcohol syndrome. I mentally reviewed several such syndromes and felt that Damien's normal appearance excluded them.

Just before beginning the worksheets, Damien had met with our psychologist Debra Fisher, who elicited details of Damien's home life. I flipped through the report. Damien denied any ongoing physical or sexual abuse, and asserted that his mother and father had a "nice" marriage. I particularly liked Debra since she had a very accepting way of asking questions. She'd say something like, "Many boys your age have friends who drink alcohol, and this is something we just ask about. Have you ever been to a party or event where people drank alcohol?" She'd then ask if Damien had ever felt pressured to drink alcohol, and finally if he himself had ever drank. In such a manner, she'd intensify her exploration of Damien's high-risk behaviors, gradually asking about smoking, marijuana, and other drugs, and then move to discuss his sexual behavior. (This approach is highly effective in getting people to discuss their personal lives. In 1993, I wrote a health survey administered by the Kentucky Department of Health to a large sample of state residents. In a stepwise fashion, a portion of the survey asked about domestic violence, beginning with "Have you ever had a verbal argument with your partner?" and culminating with "Have you ever been beaten by your partner?" About 10 percent of women admitted being seen in an emergency room for injuries inflicted by a domestic partner.)

Based on Debra's report, Damien's school problems couldn't be blamed on substance abuse or household chaos. His hearing and vision tests were normal, which ruled out simple myopia or

deafness. A careful physical exam showed no evidence of serious illness like thyroid disease. Routine blood tests by his pediatrician had
ruled out any lead poisoning or anemia. Now, a developmental specialist and I observed Tamika perform a series of "neurodevelop-
mental" tests on Damien. Through these tests, we tried to get a sense
of how Damien's mind worked: Did he have trouble reading or pro-
cessing written language? Was his hand-eye coordination normal?
How was his long-term and short-term memory? Was he easily
frustrated by complex tasks? Behind the one-way mirror, I watched
for about an hour as Tamika completed the tests, which are part of a
commercially available program. I scored the items as Damien finished them. He was particularly good at remembering and repeat-
ing a complex series of hand movements, but was fairly poor at
figuring out how a set of shapes could interlock to form a specific
design. Similarly, he was exceptionally facile at tapping separate
rhythms with his hands simultaneously, but was unable to summa-
rize the key points of a story told to him. By the end of the hour, I
had a pretty good sense of Damien's academic strengths and weak-
nesses.

Unlike the children of Garrison Keillor's beloved Lake Wobegon,
who are "all above average," children in reality have widely distributed mental and physical traits. To appreciate how this complicates
the diagnosis of learning disabilities, let's consider height. Suppose
we take one hundred previously healthy eleven-year-old boys, measure them, and compute an average, or "mean," height. This is about
56 inches. Now let's line up the boys in order of height, from short-
est to tallest. We will likely find that the middle boys are about 56
inches tall. About two-thirds of the boys fall within two inches of
the average height; thus, two inches is the "standard deviation." A
statistical property of many traits such as height is that 95 percent
of a population falls within two standard deviations of the mean.
Thus, only five boys in our hypothetical group will be either shorter
than 52 inches or taller than 60 inches. Does, then, an eleven-year-

old boy over 60 inches tall have a medical condition? We really don't know. He may have a problem with the pituitary gland, like Laurie Manygoats had, but more likely he does not. *No matter what trait is measured, 5 percent of people have to be outside the mean by two standard deviations.* Thus, 5 percent of children have spatial orientation skills that are two standard deviations away from average. The same goes for short-term memory, long-term memory, and so on.

Because there is no brain scan or blood test to diagnose a learning disability, low intelligence, dyslexia, and other problems are defined not by clear biological criteria but by statistical parameters. This is a curious diagnostic situation. For example, people with an IQ score two standard deviations below the mean are generally labeled "mentally retarded." Children who perform poorly on a certain standardized test are deemed to have a medical condition, such as reading dyslexia. But, for example, when a doctor must explain exactly what "reading dyslexia" means in a biological sense, a silence usually results. Psychologist Edwin Boring showed the tautological nature of these definitions in 1923. "Intelligence," he declared, "is what the intelligence test measures."

Because learning disabilities are defined statistically, a determined person who subjects a child to enough testing may eventually find one. For any given test, there is a 2.5 percent chance that one will fall two standard deviations below the mean. Thus, a child subjected to a battery of tests measuring twenty independent types of learning abilities has a 40 percent chance, based on statistical probability alone, of being deficient in at least one area. He can thus be diagnosed with a "learning disability" and perhaps get a coveted IEP guaranteeing extra attention from teachers or counselors.

Increasingly, I saw the whole industry of diagnosing learning disabilities as an advocacy program for children run by pediatricians. If schools had smaller class sizes and adequate resources, perhaps our intervention would be required less frequently. But in today's educational system of limited means, we draw attention to children who required a little extra help. At least, that's how I rationalized my diagnoses and recommendations for many children with very mild problems.

But then there were also children like Damien who had something truly disabling. While Damien worked with Tamika, he incessantly bounced his legs up and down. He seemed very easily distracted; when Tamika turned her head for just a second, Damien immediately got up to examine a red ball left in the corner. Another time, he deserted Tamika midsentence to run to the window, where a fire engine passed on the street. He seemed driven by a motor, which idled as he sat in his chair and was instantly thrown into gear at any opportunity. For me, he passed what Leon Gordis, the former chief of epidemiology at Johns Hopkins, called the "intra-ocular test." In contrast to complex statistical analysis, the intra-ocular test is pretty simple: if something hits you between the eyes, it must be significant. A set of questionnaires completed by Damien's parents and teachers were scored and confirmed my impression: he had attention deficit with hyperactivity disorder, or ADHD.

To appreciate what it's like to have ADHD, imagine the brain is a busy airport where many thoughts, represented by airplanes, are continuously coming and going. Just as an air traffic controller supervises the taking off and landing of flights from the runway, the brain's "executive center" coordinates the entry and exit of thoughts from consciousness. To prevent chaos, a controller must decide which flights are urgent, and which ones may wait. By prioritizing the traffic of planes, she ensures that the airport is organized. Similarly, the executive center allows thoughts to be processed in an organized fashion. A child who knows an answer to a teacher's question raises his hand, waits to be called on, stands up, and recites the answer. In the child with ADHD, the air traffic controller of his mind is absent. The child may jump from his seat and yell the answer to a question without being called upon. He may take something from a classmate without asking. He may, in short, act like Damien.

The treatment of ADHD has been studied since 1937. Working at the Emma Bradley Home in Rhode Island that year with a grant from the Supreme Council of Masons, psychiatrist Charles Bradley decided to try a drug called Benzedrine on thirty children in his hospital. In Germany, L. Edeleano had synthesized the compound some fifty years earlier, by combining an organic acid (benzoic acid) with an extract of the herb ephedra (ephedrine), creating the first member of a class of drugs later called amphetamines. The effects of Benzedrine on mood intrigued Bradley, who decided without any informed consent to try an experiment. The thirty children of "normal" intelligence he tested suffered from a variety of conditions, including "a retiring schizoid child on the one hand and the aggressive, egocentric epileptic child on the other." Bradley found that upon getting a morning dose of Benzedrine,

> fourteen children responded in spectacular fashion. Different teachers, reporting on these patients, who varied in age and school accomplishment, agreed that a great increase of interest in school material was noted immediately. There appeared a definite "drive" to accomplish as much as possible during the school period, and often to spend extra time completing additional work.

In later years, scores of studies on the use of amphetamines in children with "hyperkinesis" or "minimal brain dysfunction"—old terms for ADHD—found that roughly 75 percent improved when given amphetamines, demonstrating better concentration, school achievement, and behavior. This is higher than the not insignificant 39 percent improvement noted when these children were given placebos, implying either that a third of children with ADHD spontaneously improve, or that the pills have a strong placebo effect.

Should Damien thus be treated with stimulants? Much has been made of the so-called overprescription of stimulant medications such as methylphenidate (sold under the brand name Ritalin) or various amphetamines (sold under, among others, the brand names Dexedrine and Adderal). Drug Enforcement Administration production quotas for methylphenidate manufacturers increased from 1,768 kilograms in 1990 to 10,410 kilograms in 1995. In Maryland, which tracks statewide treatment statistics for children with ADHD, about 3 percent of schoolchildren received medication in 1995, which is a sixfold increase from 1971.

Deciding if ADHD is today overtreated or appropriately treated is a complex proposition. First, one must define what symptoms constitute ADHD. The *Diagnostic and Statistical Manual of Mental Disorders* defines all currently known psychiatric disorders, and it requires the following features to diagnose ADHD of the hyperactive variety: presence of at least six specific symptoms of hyperactivity, onset before the age of seven years, symptoms in two or more settings such as home and school, evidence of impairment of daily living or school function, and the absence of other psychiatric problems as the full explanation of the symptoms. In the late 1980s, studies in the United States estimated that 6 to 7 percent of *all* children met this definition. When compared to normal children, those with ADHD are arrested four times more frequently then normal children, fail school more often, and develop alcoholism and drug problems more frequently. Based on this data, one even could argue that ADHD is *under*diagnosed today, and children are suffering from our lack of vigilance.

However, no one knows whether the *correct* children are diagnosed with ADHD. The majority of children evaluated for ADHD see only a pediatrician and not a set of psychologists and developmental specialists as Damien did. In contrast to our evaluation of Damien, which lasted four hours and cost $1,200, the average visit where ADHD is diagnosed lasts only thirty-eight minutes and is billable at only one-tenth of our fee. Less than two-thirds of providers take the time to use the fairly reliable teacher questionnaires like the ones we used for Damien to diagnose ADHD. Instead, most pediatricians rely on a general impression of the child's behavior in the office and a parent's history. This is a risky practice; one study showed that parent reports of their child's behavior in school were very different than teacher reports. In this setting, therefore, perhaps some pediatricians simply give stimulant pills without properly finding out why children are failing at school.

Getting back to Damien, we decided he would benefit from a trial of methylphenidate. We also prescribed specific behavior therapy for Damien. As recommended by the American Academy of Pediatrics in 2001, behavior therapy is an effective adjunct to medications. Damien's parents were advised to attend a class once weekly for eight weeks to learn how to cope with a child with ADHD. Damien's teacher should ideally utilize a reward system for good behavior (using points or tokens), give feedback to Damien's parents with a daily report card, and have immediate feedback (verbal praise or time-outs) for good or bad behavior in class. Damien should also continue his weekly therapy with the school counselor. As with any chronic illness, successful management of ADHD requires a lot of work from the child and the adults who care for him.

Briefly, I reviewed other therapies for ADHD. In 1974, the allergist Ben Feingold claimed in his influential book *Why Your Child Is Hyperactive* that artificial foods, colors, and flavoring were responsible for half of all cases of ADHD. Although later studies didn't support the scope of Feingold's claim, some found that removal of the preservative tartrazine and foods causing allergy sometimes may help some children with ADHD. I take a parent's concerns about food seriously; however, Damien's mother didn't report any special sensitivity. Although some children are better focused when listening to music (audiotherapy), there is no evidence to support homeopathy, vision therapy, megavitamin use, or restricting sugar and aspartame (Nutrasweet).

Damien returned to see us one month afterward. His improvement was substantial. Behind the one-way mirror, I noted how he seemed to sit more still, without shaking his legs constantly. Though his attention wandered occasionally, Damien completed his testing with increased focus. He had made a new friend at school, who was coming over later that day. Damien's mother confirmed our impression. The reports from school were improved, and her son's impulsiveness had decreased. She was enjoying him more at home, without getting into battles with him as frequently. She said to us, "Thank you for giving my child back to me." We arranged for follow-up in about two months to reassess Damien's performance.

Though their effect was dramatic, stimulant medications will never cure Damien. Multiple studies have shown that while the drugs help in the short term, they don't fix the problem long term. In an erudite review of many studies on the prognosis of children with ADHD, Russel Barkley wrote in 1976, "Stimulant drugs appear to facilitate management of the hyperkinetic children but do not provide the necessary influence to alter later social and academic adjustment." To help a child get through school, the drugs furnish a dimly lit tunnel. The child must learn to light his own way brightly, because the darkness will never fully dissipate. Most affected children continue having symptoms of ADHD into adulthood.

I explained this to the family. As Damien left after his visit, I silently wished him courage. Despite his mother's ebullience, we hadn't really cured him.

~ 6 ~

Skin

ON THE MAKING AND BREAKING OF CONTACT

After removing his shirt in the Newborn Intensive Care Unit, Adam's father sat back on a recliner next to his premature son's isolette. A few times the size of a breadbox, an isolette is a Plexiglas incubator used to keep premature infants warm while in the hospital. The isolette was necessary for two reasons. First, the part of Adam's brain that regulates body temperature, the thermoregulation center in the hypothalamus, was not yet fully developed. Second, Adam needed all his energy to grow, and leaving him in the open air would require expending precious calories to stay warm rather than to gain much-needed weight.

I met Adam's father, a husky man named Paul, for the first time in the delivery room where his wife gave birth to twins by cesarean section. Although normal gestation takes about forty weeks, Adam and his twin were born prematurely after only thirty-two weeks and required the resuscitation measures described in the chapter about lungs. Now almost one week old, Adam lay sleeping in the isolette.

Though Paul sat bare-chested in the NICU, no one thought this was unusual. A nurse removed little Adam from the isolette and took off his hospital jumper, leaving the newborn wearing only a diaper. She then placed Adam belly down on top of Paul's chest, so that father and son were joined skin to skin. Finally, she covered Adam's body with a cotton blanket. Paul leaned back in the recliner and closed his eyes.

Mimicking a practice of marsupials, Paul was engaged in "kangaroo positioning." A component of what is today termed Kangaroo Maternal Care, or KMC, this skin-to-skin method of keeping an infant warm was developed at a Bogotá, Colombia, hospital in 1978 in response to economic and manpower shortages at a newborn unit. Marsupials like kangaroos and possums are all born prematurely, and since their gestational development is incomplete the newborn is unable to survive if separated physically from the mother. The marsupial child completes its development in the mother's pouch, where it is kept warm and nursed with breast milk. Unable to access enough isolettes for premature infants, the Bogotá hospital adapted this behavior. Mothers were asked to room-in with their babies and practice KMC, which included continuous skin-to-skin contact and exclusive breast-feeding. In an experience widely publicized by UNICEF, the hospital found excellent rates of survival and great satisfaction among mothers. Today kangaroo positioning is practiced at many modern NICU facilities, which find it an ideal way to promote bonding between parent and child while still allowing the child to maintain a normal body temperature outside its isolette.

Measuring body temperature is a relatively modern undertaking. Though Heron of Alexandria had developed an instrument measuring thermal changes with a column of water in the second century, modern thermometry wasn't invented until 1714 when Gabriel Fahrenheit began using mercury in a sealed cylinder. This let scientists make objective and reproducible measurements. Until then, a person with "fever" was understood to have a quickened pulse, subjective chills, weakness, and only incidentally an elevated body temperature. With the benefit of Fahrenheit's device, Herman Boerhaave suggested that an elevated temperature was the critical finding in fever. This hypothesis led Carl Wunderlich in Germany to study comprehensively the distribution of body temperature in a seminal 1868 monograph, for which he took almost two million body temperatures and concluded that 98.6 degrees Fahrenheit was average. Though a belief in this standard survives today (the 1990 edition of *Stedman's Medical Dictionary* defines fever as "a bodily temperature above the normal of 98.6°F"), average body temperature is actually closer to 98.2 degrees according to more recent studies. A person is warmest in the late afternoon and coolest in the early morning by about half a degree. Since it was about 4 P.M., little Adam was perched on skin that was warmed to about 99 degrees Fahrenheit.

The brain controls body temperature much like a thermostat regulates a house's temperature. Small nerves in skin measure temperature and transmit this information to the thermoregulation center in the brain. There, the skin temperature is compared to the brain's desired temperature, or setpoint. If the skin temperature is too high, then the body's cooling system is activated. Blood vessels on the skin dilate, so the body loses heat like a car dissipates heat through the radiator. Sweat glands release up to a liter of coolant onto the skin. Finally a person breathes faster, which chills the body since the inhaled air is colder than body temperature.

When the body temperature is lower than the setpoint, the body's heating system is turned on. Blood vessels on the skin constrict to prevent heat loss through convection, and a person may shiver to produce heat. In infants, the brain also activates the body's natural furnace and consumes oil. Normal infants have two types of fat: brown and white. If white fat cells can be likened to a down comforter on a bed, then brown fat cells are an electric blanket. Located near the shoulders and also near the heart and kidneys, brown fat cells split oil apart to produce heat, in response to signals from the brain.

For Adam, the isolette assumed the task of maintaining body temperature. In addition to his brain's immaturity, Adam lacked substantial brown fat stores (to generate heat) and white fat in the skin (to contain heat). A small gold-foil sensor in the shape of a heart glued to Adam's belly read his skin temperature and transmitted it to the isolette. We inputted the setpoint for Adam's body on a digital panel on the isolette. When Adam was cooler than the setpoint, the isolette pumped warm air to Adam until he was the right temperature. As the Bogotá researchers found, this could also be done naturally without a complex electronic machine.

In the recliner, Paul performed the same function. When Adam was placed on his father's chest, he essentially became an appendage of Paul's body. Lying there, a father was connected to his son not just emotionally but also physiologically. If Adam got colder than his father, Paul's skin conducted heat to his skin to warm him. In the process, Paul's skin got slightly colder and in response the hypothalamus activated Paul's internal warming system. In this manner, Adam was warmed to about 99 degrees.

An investment banker, Paul showed up at the NICU after work every day to "kangaroo" Adam for about forty minutes. Because he couldn't easily talk on a telephone, read business materials, or write while his son lay on his chest, Paul said that he thought a lot about his life. It was a meditative experience. Perhaps he was working too hard and not spending time with his wife. He promised that things would be different this time. As a medical student on an oncology rotation years earlier, I noted that many patients with critical illness expressed regret that they hadn't spent more time with their families—an observation remarkable for both its triteness and instructiveness. Perhaps after his experiences in the NICU, Paul would change his priorities.

Next to Adam's isolette, another child, Jack, was struggling to stay alive. A "micro-preemie," Jack weighed only two pounds and was born at twenty-five weeks of gestation—only six months. He was critically ill. In addition to his other problems, this infant couldn't maintain his temperature despite being in an isolette. This child was placed on a radiant warmer, which is a table with heating lamps like those used at fast-food restaurants to keep food warm. On the table, Saran wrap was stretched over the child because his skin hadn't developed enough to contain heat as well as Adam's.

The body's largest organ, the skin develops in stages beginning in the first month after conception. In a fully developed child, the skin is composed of several layers beginning with the deepest one, the dermis, and ending at the outermost layer, the epidermis. Jack was born so early that several key layers were lacking. His skin was transparent, and one could see blood vessels below it. So amorphous that it's termed "gelatinous," the skin was unable to insulate Jack. Kangaroo positioning is not effective for such infants. Jack's parents sat in silence next to the radiant warmer, and his mother touched him through the Saran wrap with a finger.

At one point, I saw Paul glance over at this unfortunate child and clutch his own son closer. He then closed his eyes and returned to his thoughts.

Skin packages organs into bodies. It protects us from infections, water loss, and excessive ultraviolet radiation. The skin also synthesizes a key nutrient, vitamin D, when exposed to the sun. And as just described, skin determines our temperature. Comprising almost a fifth of body weight, the skin processes our tactile interactions with the world. Among organs it is a celebrity, displayed publicly and lavished with the most extravagant attentions. We use moisturizers, razors, perfumes, mud, salves, and soaps to beautify skin since people notice its colors, texture, and imperfections. Because skin is so visible, many parents quickly find out if something is wrong with their baby's skin, and bring the child to see a pediatrician. That's how I met one-week-old Daria Ringer.

Daria's mother was concerned that the baby had developed a diaper rash and that her usual creams weren't helping. This was a common complaint at our clinic in Gallup, New Mexico.

First described in 1921 as an "ammoniacal scald," diaper rash occurs in about one in five infants, most commonly around one year of age. Interestingly, the rash is caused by a combination of both urine and stool, and not by either one alone. Enzymes called ureases found in stool conspire with urine to produce an elevated pH around the buttocks. This pH increase activates substances called lipases and proteases in stool, which actually digest the skin around the buttock and cause the irritating rash so familiar to parents.

The widespread adoption of disposable diapers in the 1970s decreased rates of diaper rash. As science journalist Malcolm Gladwell delicately points out, the typical child's "insult" shoots into a diaper at about a tablespoon's worth in two seconds, or an ounce every four seconds. The average insult lasts ten seconds. A wonder of modern technology, today's superabsorbent diapers can withstand three such insults and still leave the baby's bottom dry. Though they occupy almost 2 percent of American landfill space, disposable diapers have saved many baby buttocks from erosion. Daria's parents used a common brand of superabsorbent diaper.

Still, many infants develop diaper rashes anyway. When an over-the-counter occlusive paste like zinc oxide fails to cure the rash, it's likely that a fungus called *Candida* has infected the wound. Thus, doctors prescribe the same type of lotion used for athlete's foot or vaginal yeast infections to heal the baby's skin. That's what Daria's pediatrician initially suspected the problem was. But when he removed Daria's diaper, it was clear that the child had no ordinary diaper rash.

On the baby's left buttock, a dime-sized area of skin was ulcerated and looked like raw hamburger meat. Whereas ordinary diaper rashes can cause a small amount of skin breakdown, this lesion was much more serious. There are rare diseases in which infants fail to absorb zinc from breast milk or lack the ability to process a B-complex vitamin called biotin. Such infants develop a persistent diaper rash that doesn't respond to conventional therapy, but Daria's erosion was deeper than the lesions usually found in these conditions. Daria's pediatrician, Jason Liddy, thus admitted her to the hospital for further management. He didn't know what the problem was, and thought we could observe its progress better in the hospital. I first saw Daria the day after her admission, when Jason signed out her care to me for the weekend because I was on call.

Jason was easy to identify; he was well over six feet tall and sported a shaved head. The skin of his scalp shone like a beacon. Like myself, he moved to Navajo country a year earlier from what the locals called "out East." But we were quite different from each other. Before medical school he had attended a Jesuit seminary and taken a vow of chastity. He arose daily at four o'clock to read medical journals and religious scripture, and then worked out at a local gym called Wowie's for two hours before work. Well muscled, Jason supplemented his diet—despite the ridicule of our entire practice— with various protein shakes. In contrast, I hadn't attended any religious school and consider myself an agnostic. I wake up a half hour before work and barely make it to the hospital on time. Needless to say, no fancy bodybuilding cocktails have ever passed through my lips.

But we're connected by a common practice style. Many physicians inhabit distinct personal and professional spheres; your personality in a certain area often belies your personality in the other. Although Jason and I share almost nothing in common outside the wards, we practice medicine like doppelgangers. We each pore over medical literature with the earnestness of Talmudic scholars, often see eye to eye on the management of complicated illnesses, and are energized when asked to explain and defend our medical decisions during rounds. We enjoy the dynamic nature of medical practice, the constant struggle to refine the care we provide.

Medical knowledge is continually progressing. In an effort to promote continued education, states require licensed physicians periodically to furnish evidence that they have regularly attended educational conferences or taken courses to update their knowledge base. Theoretically, these measures should ensure that all doctors practice according to the most recent standards. Unfortunately, the reality is much different. Scores of studies looking at conference attendance, printed handout distribution, financial incentives, and chart audits by reviewers all tell the same story: most physicians are mulelike in their stubbornness to update their practices, no matter how out of date they may be. That's why I was happy to work with Jason, as few physicians like learning as much as he does.

Jason and I entered Daria's room. The child's parents weren't around, and she was sleeping on her belly. Jason and I removed her diaper while she slept and examined her skin. "I'm treating it like a burn," said Jason. Twice daily, an ointment called Silvadene was applied to the area, and the bandages were changed. "It seems worse today," admitted Jason. 'What do you think we should do next?"

The truth was, neither of us knew for sure. A little secret of advanced medical care is that—even for the most up-to-date doctors around—most of it is based on limited or nonexistent evidence. In a publicized 1978 report, the U.S. Office of Technology Assessment concluded, "Only 10% to 20% of all procedures currently used in medical practice have been shown to be efficacious by controlled trial." More recently, a 1999 British study found that only 40 percent of pediatric care is supported by high-quality data. Surprisingly, most of what we doctors do has never been proven effective. One could say that we're largely selling snake oil—that is, *expensive* snake oil—under the guise of science.

But this characterization is overly harsh. The frequent absence of hard data produces uncertainty, but also creates an art to medicine. Relying on intuition and experience, a doctor must choose among several reasonable treatments. In Daria's case, there was no single recipe for healing a raw buttock ulcer. We had many options. We could treat the wound as a burn and continue the dressing care. Perhaps then the wound would heal with time. Or we could assume that given the wound's location, its repeated contamination by defecation explained why the skin wasn't healing. If this were the case, we'd recommend a colostomy, a temporary redirection of her large intestine so that stool came out of her abdomen. Or perhaps we'd use immune-boosting drugs, because Daria might have a defect in her immune system that made it difficult for her to heal a simple diaper rash.

When making any important medical decision with limited information, it's best to start with the most benign treatment and assess a patient frequently. That way, if the patient is getting better you've spared her from toxic therapies, and if the patient gets sicker you have something stronger to try. Jason and I agreed to continue the benign Silvadene ointment for another day and see if the lesion healed. We recommended she be positioned belly-down on a pillow, with her bare buttocks raised into the air. Leaving her exposed in open air decreased any chance that moisture would accumulate around the wound and worsen the skin breakdown.

Our plan didn't work. The next day, Daria's buttock looked worse; what had previously been dime-sized was now the diameter of a quarter. Daria seemed miserable from her unnatural positioning. Jason and I regrouped at her bedside the next morning. "It's expanding," he agreed.

We resumed our discussion where we'd left off the day earlier. Jason opened, "Maybe we're dealing with a group A streptococcal infection. You know, flesh-eating bacteria." I shook my head. "Her condition is too indolent for that. There's no fever, spreading erythema, or lymphangitis. I don't think it's infected." Jason smiled; he was just warming up. He countered, "What about a toxin?"

Was it possible? A year earlier, I'd been called to the emergency room because a two-year-old girl in Window Rock, Arizona, walked into her backyard and startled a rattlesnake. It bit her big toe. By the time she arrived to the hospital, her leg was swollen massively and the skin near the bite had begun to ulcerate. Rattlesnake venom is superbly adapted to destroying skin and spreading itself. Enzymes called proteases and hyaluronidases first digest the skin near the bite in a related but more powerful fashion than those that cause diaper rash. (This likely evolved because snakes can't chew their prey; the venom predigests their victims.) Then, the venom commandeers the immune system by causing the release of histamine from certain white blood cells. In a normal person, histamine increases the permeability of blood vessels near an infection, so that immune cells can leave the bloodstream and arrive where they're needed. Rattlesnake venom ingeniously reverses this process, allowing its transport from the now-soupy skin wound into the bloodstream. Then the mischief really starts: the venom busts apart red blood cells, interferes with clotting, and, in some cases, paralyzes the victim.

I'd never forget that night, having spent five hours in the pharmacy mixing up antivenin by hand for the toddler. After getting the antidote, the girl ended up doing well. Invented in 1954 and commonly called "Wyeth serum" after its manufacturer, the antivenin itself carried a small risk of inducing a fatal allergic reaction. But it also reduces the risk of death from about 20 percent to about 1 percent. (Recently, Wyeth-Ayerst announced it would no longer make this antivenin; a new one called CroFab with fewer side effects was approved for use in the United States.) Antivenins are really the only effective treatment for rattlesnake bites. Tying a tourniquet around the bitten limb, cutting open the wound, and sucking it by mouth are nonsense that may worsen the problem.

Jason had a valid point when he mentioned a toxin. A bite— from a venomous snake or even a brown recluse spider—could cause an ulcer that didn't heal with our treatment. But I pointed out that Daria couldn't have survived a rattlesnake bite without treatment. Plus, it seemed far-fetched that a rattlesnake bit Daria on the buttock without her parents noticing. Similarly, a spider would have bitten her arms or legs, not her buttock, which was covered by a diaper. "I don't think it's a toxin," I said to Jason. Somewhat mischievously, I asked, "What about an obscure immune deficiency like Job syndrome? "

But I failed to confound him. After all, he was a Jesuit scholar who'd certainly understand the allusion in the syndrome's moniker. Technically known as hypergammaglobulin E syndrome, the ailment derives its common name from the biblical character tested by a lifelong affliction of draining skin infections. "Impossible," Jason answered with a smile. "Too young for presentation. And don't even think about leukocyte adhesion disorder." Jason referred to the rare immune problem whose hallmark is that the umbilical cord doesn't fall off a newborn in time. Children with this disease have poor skin healing, and occasionally develop boils on the buttocks.

We continued this repartee for another few minutes without developing an airtight theory to explain Daria's problem. In the absence of consensus, we decided to continue the Silvadene and reassess the next day. Unfortunately, the ulcer became even bigger, now the size of a half-dollar. We were definitely missing something.

In the meantime, Daria's parents hadn't visited since their baby's admission. The poor girl lay facedown with her buttocks raised up and spent most of the day crying. I wondered why her parents didn't feel enough connection to Daria to visit. In the late 1960s, psychiatrist

John Bowlby developed a framework called attachment theory, which hypothesized that all people have a need to form affectional bonds with others. Inspired by the studies of Konrad Lorenz who demonstrated that newborn geese could be "imprinted" to believe a human was their parent, Bowlby sought to understand the determinants of human bonding. He postulated that normal attachment begins shortly after birth, and its development depends on reciprocity. For example, when an infant smiles, clings to a parent, or cries, an adult responds by smiling back, holding the baby, or offering food. As another psychologist later summarized, "The experience of security is the goal of the attachment system, which is a regulator of emotional experience." In other words, reciprocity leads to feelings of security, which are critical for an infant's normal development. What, then, might happen to Daria if her parents didn't show up when she cried, didn't soothe her with their touch, and weren't the ones who fed her?

The consequences of neglect, if prolonged, can be severe. In the 1970s, Mary Ainsworth developed a laboratory procedure called the "Strange Situation" to study infants' attachment. One- to two-year-old infants were briefly separated from their parents in an unfamiliar room and their reactions recorded. Ainsworth found four distinct patterns. Well-attached infants, termed "secure," were distressed by parent absence momentarily, but returned to their regular activities when the parent returned. "Anxious/avoidant" infants didn't seem to mind that the parent had left, and didn't seem to notice when the parent returned. "Anxious/resistant" children showed unusual distress (such as screaming and persistent crying), which improved very slowly after the parent returned. Finally, a group of infants was "disorganized/disoriented," showing head-banging, temporary paralysis, and unusual avoidance of unfamiliar situations when left alone. In particular, these last infants often had suffered sexual or physical abuse, prolonged separation from parents, or intense marital conflict between parents. These infants are hard to rehabilitate, since numerous long-term studies suggest that three-quarters of people maintain the same attachment classification from infancy to adulthood. Most worrisome, people classified as "disorganized/disoriented" are at high risk of psychopathology in later life. That's why I worried about Daria.

Unfortunately, detaching from their children is how some parents deal with guilt or loss. Recently I was called to a delivery where a newborn had mild breathing trouble. By the time I arrived, the distress had resolved and the child was fine. Strangely, the mother was recuperating in a separate wing of the hospital. I went to her room to reassure her, and she listened with a hard look on her face. "Do you want to see your girl?" I asked. "I don't want to see her," she responded, coldly. For a moment I lost my objectivity, and blurted, "But she's your child. Why not?" She repeated, "I don't want to see her," and motioned me to the door. I later learned the baby was being given up; her mother had a history of serial child neglect rooted in her alcoholism. The labor nurse described how the mother had cried out during the delivery, not about her physical pain but about her powerlessness against alcohol. By never seeing her daughter, the mother insulated herself from an attachment that would only be destroyed by her addiction.

Other conditions like postpartum depression and major birth defects or illness also alienate parents from their newborns. But Daria's parents had no known addictions, mental health problems, or history of child neglect, and a buttock ulcer didn't seem like a horrific illness. Since they had no phone on the reservation, Jason and I dealt with their absence by leaving daily messages with their relatives. We hoped they'd show up sometime soon and have a good excuse.

"We need to send her to a burn unit," Jason told me after we examined Daria that morning. With their specialized wound care, such a center might have better luck. After all, we were in an isolated setting with no plastic surgeons or specially trained wound-care nurses. A wise physician knows when to give up a patient, just as a good basketball player must pass off the ball when he's cornered. We made some calls and handed off Daria to an Albuquerque tertiary care center.

A few days later, we received a call from a surgeon involved in Daria's care. At first her case was perplexing, he said. The team caring for Daria continued the wound care begun in Gallup with only minor changes. The ulcer didn't worsen, but it didn't improve either. Soon afterward, they noticed something very interesting: some edges of the wound developed a reddish tinge. Over the next few days, this beachhead expanded until it surrounded the initial wound. This red ring resembled the surface of a strawberry and grew to a centimeter wide around the ulcer.

Daria's problem suddenly became clear, and I felt foolish for having missed it earlier. About two years ago, I had given an introductory lecture at Children's Hospital in Boston before the main speaker, Judah Folkman, described his groundbreaking work on what I suddenly realized was also Daria's problem.

A former chief of pediatric surgery, Folkman has an unassuming demeanor that belies his position as one of the most influential researchers at Children's Hospital today. As a medical student he developed a novel method of repairing a pediatric heart defect and was the first student ever invited to address the American College of Surgery. He graduated at the top of his class at Harvard Medical School and completed his training in surgery at Massachusetts General Hospital. Soon afterward, Folkman decided to challenge a fundamental assumption about the growth of tumors. Traditionally, surgeons believed that tumors grew in size, followed blood vessels, invaded them, and then spread through the body. Folkman instead proposed that tumors grew their own blood vessels; that is, a tumor made its own infrastructure to nourish itself. This was a heretical notion. Praising this audacity, Bill Speck, the director of the famed Marine Biological Laboratories, later said that Folkman had "to see what everyone has seen and to think what nobody has thought." By identifying the substances made by tumors that controlled the growth of blood vessels—termed angiogenesis factors—Folkman proved his contention. Folkman then synthesized angiogenesis *inhibitors,* or chemicals that prevent the growth of blood vessels, which are today hailed as a silver bullet that may cure numerous cancers by destroying their supply lines.

Folkman's work had critical significance for Daria. Almost one in three newborns have birthmarks called "stork bites" or "angel kisses," which are actually very small tumors of blood vessels on the surface of the skin. They typically disappear after a few months. But in some children the birthmark can grow for six to twelve months, and eventually resembles a strawberry sitting on the skin. This is called a hemangioma. Just as mysteriously as it appears, the hemangioma then melts away and is completely gone in most children by six years of age. Folkman realized that natural angiogenesis factors and inhibitors regulate this waxing and waning.

In a small subset of children, hemangiomas don't regress and instead continue to grow, sometimes to the size of a grapefruit. This can be a vision- or life-threatening condition if the hemangioma occurs on the face, eyes, or within a vital organ like the lungs. In 1988, Folkman received a call from Carl White of Denver, a physician caring for a child with hemangiomas that were frequently bleeding. The usual treatment, steroids, had failed and the child would likely die of the illness without an effective intervention. Folkman proposed giving the child an angiogenesis inhibitor called interferon alfa-2a, and over the next year the hemangiomas shrank. Encouraged by the result, Folkman convened a larger study proving that this result was reproducible. Today, Folkman's medicine is used regularly to treat lesions like Daria's.

Daria had a hemangioma on her buttock that was very close to the skin surface, and therefore as delicate as a spiderweb. By the time Jason and I first saw it, the strawberry vessels had been scraped from contact with the diaper, and only an ulcer was left. That's why we missed the diagnosis. However, the tumor grew so quickly that it eventually surpassed the margin of the ulcer it was causing and was able to be identified. To put it simply, Daria's problem was a birthmark that grew out of control.

The surgeon from Albuquerque mentioned that Daria's parents had visited a few times. They hadn't come to our hospital because of car problems, they had told him. In Albuquerque, Daria's mother clearly was invested in her daughter, and she learned how to change the dressings and clean the wound carefully. Because the ulcer appeared to be healing, the plan now was to discharge Daria, have her mother perform the dressing changes for two weeks, and then reassess the wound. If it continued to grow and ulcerate, an angiogenesis inhibitor might be necessary. If it kept healing, we'd just continue the dressing changes.

Two weeks later, Daria returned to see us in Gallup after her discharge. We placed her on the exam table, removed her diaper, and peeled back the dressing. The wound really did look better. Instead of resembling hamburger, the ulcer had a mayonnaise-textured coating called granulation tissue.

A healing wound, or scar, can be likened to a commercial construction project. After skin is damaged, a blood clot forms and white blood cells drift through the area to clear debris. Then, like workers pouring a foundation, cells called fibroblasts lay down material called collagen. The wound is now said to be "granulating," like Daria's scar. Lending tensile strength, cells called myofibroblasts pull the edges of the scar together, just as steel rods are tightened to support a building's foundation. Deep within the skin, basal cells then divide, erecting a column of cells to restore the skin's integrity. Finally keratin, the capstone of the skin, is placed. Healing is then complete, although minor changes in skin color and tone can continue for several months. During this time, pediatricians recommend shielding the scar from prolonged sunlight and occasionally using vitamin E lotions (their efficacy is controversial) to ensure that the skin returns to normal.

Daria wouldn't require an angiogenesis inhibitor, since the hemangioma was already regressing on its own. Her mother, a silent woman from the western part of the reservation, allowed a slight smile when we told her this. She then opened a leather satchel and extracted a shiny tube of ointment and a new surgical dressing for Daria. Then she carefully applied the ointment just as the Albuquerque surgeons had taught her. Watching her, I imagined the myofibroblasts pulling through collagen, strengthening the connection between the wound's edges. Daria's mother applied the gauze over the ointment and taped it down expertly. Then she hoisted the girl into her arms, covered her with a colorful shawl, and walked slowly out of the room.

"Could you please take a look at a child?" a nurse urgently asked me in the emergency room at Children's Hospital. I nodded and followed her. We stopped outside a room with a heavy wooden door. Opening it and entering the anteroom, the nurse donned a gown, yellow gloves, and a microfilter face mask. I followed suit. We proceeded through another door into the isolation room, where a five-year-old boy named Patrick Powell lay on a bed. Looking drained, his father dozed in an adjacent chair.

I flipped through the chart. The boy had a fever of 101 degrees Fahrenheit, and his heart was racing. There was a diffuse collection of spots over his trunk, arms, and legs. I looked at one of the lesions carefully. The size of an almond, the rose-colored spot was topped with a clear vesicle resembling a dewdrop. The nurse looked at me knowingly, and we woke the boy's father. "Your son," I said to him, "has chickenpox."

The name chickenpox has nothing to do with poultry; instead, it's thought to be derived from either the Old English *gican*, meaning itch, or the Old French word *chiche-pois*, meaning chickpea, thought to describe the size of the lesions. Until 1767, chickenpox and its deadlier imitator smallpox were not distinguished. The medical term for chickenpox is varicella, which is a Latin diminutive of variola, the word for smallpox. However, the causative viruses are from separate evolutionary families and have little in common.

Patrick was engaged in what has been a universal experience; 90 percent of all children younger than ten years have had chickenpox. Ninety-nine percent of adults have varicella antibodies, lingering evidence of the virus's visit. In years past, parents often saw the illness as a child's rite of passage and had parties to disseminate the infection to unexposed children. One source advised mothers to "throw a chickenpox party. . . . You can make spotty food (e.g., pancake with blueberries) and draw spotty pictures."

Patrick's father hadn't known what the spots were, and his uncertainty was understandable. A child with both fever and rash could have, at recent count, any of about fifty different infections. Historically, these conditions were named in the order they were described; for example, measles was called "first disease," scarlet fever was "second disease," German measles was "third disease," and so on up to "sixth disease," or roseola. After that, no one continued using numbers.

Some of these infections could be deadly. By far the most feared is meningococcemia, which begins innocuously with a fever and a few bruiselike marks on the body. One old-timer at Children's Hospital recalls how such a child walked into his clinic years ago, not looking too sick. Recognizing the condition, however, the doctor physically picked up the child and began sprinting from his clinic to the emergency room a few blocks away. As he ran, the child's spots, called purpura, multiplied before his eyes and the child became increasingly lethargic and passed out. That child was saved by penicillin, which snuffs out the organism if given early enough. But not all children are so lucky. A few years ago, I was the senior resident in the Children's Hospital intensive care unit when I got a call from an outside emergency room where a similar child showed up. The physician wanted to transport the child to us via helicopter, and I gave some brief medical advice and arranged the transport. Ten minutes later I called back to confirm the pickup time, and the doctor answered in a weary voice that the child had already passed away. Meningococcemia can kill that quickly.

Patrick's skin, however, was classic for chickenpox. Like the average kid, Patrick had somewhere around three hundred lesions, though they can occasionally number from only ten to over fifteen hundred. Varicella is a stealthy virus caught from particles sneezed into the air by infected children or from direct contact with their infected skin. Unknown to the host, the virus spreads into the lymph nodes four days after acquisition, and then encamps in hidden bases within the liver, spleen, and other organs. After about two weeks during which the infected child has no symptoms, the virus suddenly emerges into the bloodstream and invades the skin. Fever develops and the characteristic pox appears. Over the past two weeks, Patrick had been a broth of virus. He just didn't know it until today.

Patrick's father looked relieved when told his son had chickenpox. "So it's nothing serious, right?" he asked. I nodded, and recommended some Tylenol for the fever, cutting Patrick's fingernails, and keeping him out of school until the lesions crusted over so he wouldn't spread the contagion. In closing, his father mentioned, "I told his mother that he didn't need the new vaccine, since it's only chickenpox." Unfortunately for Jeffrey Law, a child we'll soon meet, Patrick's father expressed a common sentiment.

The vaccine is traceable to a three-year-old Japanese boy who developed chickenpox in the 1970s. Researcher Michiaki Takahashi inserted a thin needle into some of the boy's vesicles and extracted some fluid teeming with virus. Some viruses, like varicella, can be cultivated only when they have specific human cells to infect. Takahashi thus incubated the fluid with what are termed human embryonic cells, derived and cultured decades earlier from an aborted fetus. (To the consternation of many abortion foes, several vaccines, including Albert Sabin's celebrated polio vaccine, were cultivated using such cells.) Just as had been done before with smallpox, the virus was cultured and cultured until it became attenuated, that is, it lost its disease-causing ability. A person infected with this mild, attenuated strain, called Oka after its original three-year-old host's surname, was immune to the original disease-causing strain. After a decade of study, Oka was licensed for general vaccination in Japan in 1989. In the United States, Merck purchased the rights to the Oka virus and received approval in 1995 from the U.S. Food and Drug Administration to market the vaccine under the brand name Varivax.

Varivax was an immediate commercial failure. Despite recommendations from the American Academy of Pediatrics to vaccinate all susceptible children, the Centers for Disease Control estimated that only one-third of American toddlers got the vaccine in 1998, and in some states only one in twenty did.

This was so because widespread skepticism greeted Varivax after its approval. Would the vaccine last long enough to ensure that adults remained immune? Would it induce immunity in the first place? A large number of parents and physicians discounted the need for Varivax. In a 1998 letter to the New England Journal of Medicine, two doctors wrote, "[Chickenpox] has been largely a benign disease. . . . Although it is generally held that immunizing children is axiomatic for public health, vaccinating all children against chickenpox is a bad idea."

Similar opposition to vaccination existed during a 1901 epidemic of smallpox in Boston during which fifteen hundred people were infected. In response, the Boston Board of Health required that all citizens get vaccinated, or face a five-dollar fine or a fifteen-day jail sentence. Almost half a million Bostonians were vaccinated. Decrying a perceived imposition on civil rights, the Anti–Compulsory Vaccination League (which the Board of Health considered "a hotbed of the anti-vaccine heresy") protested the requirement, and the battle led to a 1905 case, *Jacobson v. Massachusetts*. The U.S. Supreme Court ruled that although the state could not mandate vaccination to protect an individual, it could do so to protect the public. This ruling also came on the heels of the publicized "Pfeiffer affair," in which the sixty-year-old physician Immanuel Pfeiffer (a former president of the American Psychic Society) tested his belief that healthy people couldn't get smallpox. After one of his bills opposing vaccination was voted down, Pfeiffer deliberately exposed himself to smallpox at a sanitarium to demonstrate his theory. He promptly became critically ill within two weeks.

There are several parallels between variola and varicella vaccine. Both induce protection in 95 percent of susceptible individuals after inoculation. The resulting immunity from both easily lasts for twenty years. Both have been rigorously studied and proven to save lives. And yet both faced social and political hurdles. Today, most people consider varicella a benign disease of no consequence, unlike smallpox, which carried a 20 to 50 percent mortality rate. Why, then, should the state require vaccination against a benign condition? The answer can be found in the case of nine-year-old Jeffrey Law. I never spoke to Jeffrey. In fact, I didn't even know his name for some time. As a second-year resident, I was a member of the code team in the emergency room. As described in the chapter about bones, the code team is assembled whenever a critically ill child is expected via ambulance. One afternoon, the call came.

The paramedics wheeled a stretcher bearing an unconscious boy into the brightly lit room. The various monitors taped to his chest beeped violently and displayed angry red numbers. The boy's breathing was shallow and he didn't respond when two nurses inserted large-bore intravenous catheters into his veins. The code leader called for silence and asked for vital signs. In clipped tones, a nurse recited, "Pulse two hundred. Blood pressure sixty over thirty. Respirations thirty. Pulse ox eighty-six percent. Temp one hundred and three." These were worrisome indeed. The fever indicated likely infection, and the rapid heart rate and poor blood pressure meant that his blood vessels were leaky and unable to hold pressure. It was as though the heart was pumping fluid through a hose riddled with holes; it didn't matter how high the spigot was turned up. This is known as "shock"—the body's misdirected response to overwhelming infection.

To fight shock, we infused liters of saline to fill the circulatory system and gave the drug dopamine to squeeze the vessels closed. Large quantities of antibiotics were injected to fight the unknown infection. Minutes after the boy arrived, the code leader asked me to perform a quick "secondary survey" of the boy's body. I pulled off the boy's shirt and, using shears, cut off his jeans. His trunk and thighs were marked with the characteristic lesions of chickenpox. The code leader nodded gravely and said, "Looks like superinfection."

The skin is usually a formidable barrier to infection. In addition to its physical armor of the protein keratin, skin has sweat glands that secrete destructive enzymes, acid, and other antibiotic substances. This is critical since a square centimeter of skin—an area smaller than a dime—teems with hundreds of thousands of bacteria like *Staphylococci*, *Bacilli*, various fungi, and *Streptococci*. When an abrasion, deep wound, or a chickenpox lesion disrupts skin, these colonizers can invade the body. The severity of infection depends on the depth of its penetration. When very superficial, the bacteria cause a mild condition called impetigo that gets better with some antibacterial ointment. When deeper, a more serious infection called cellulitis occurs, and requires treatment with oral antibiotics and occasionally hospitalization. In my patient's case, bacteria called *Streptococcus pyogenes*, the same organisms that cause strep throat, entered a chickenpox lesion and somehow made their way into the bloodstream. Because this condition involves one infection taking advantage of the opportunity created by another infection, it is termed "superinfection." The bacteria that multiplied within the boy's blood also made a poisonous toxin that increased its virulence. Hence, his condition is termed "streptococcal toxic shock syndrome."

The boy was so overwhelmed by the infection that he developed low blood pressure, which starved his body of oxygen. We barely stabilized him in the emergency room before transferring him to the intensive care unit. I saw his name on some paperwork as he was wheeled away: Jeffrey Law. Unfortunately, he died two hours later.

Chickenpox, it turns out, isn't such a harmless condition after all. At Children's Hospital, the rate of bloodstream infections linked to chickenpox tripled during the 1980s, and ten children with Jeffrey's problem were treated there in 1993. Additionally, chickenpox is linked to brain damage, pneumonia, and birth defects. In the early 1990s, varicella caused ten thousand hospitalizations per year and over one hundred deaths in the United States—more deaths than caused by all other vaccine-preventable childhood illnesses *combined.*

But the perception of chickenpox's benign nature persists. Only twenty-two states require the vaccine for school enrollment. In a 2001 survey, 50 percent of parents preferred the disease to the vaccine as a means of acquiring immunity, and 90 percent were unaware that chickenpox can kill. But when educated about the risks of varicella, 85 percent wanted vaccination for their child. Appealing to this protective instinct, Merck now markets the vaccine with a teary-eyed fowl as its mascot.

Vaccination prevents disease on a large scale only when everybody agrees to participate. In this sense, the *Jacobson v. Massachusetts* verdict was prescient indeed. Allowing individuals to refuse vaccination sacrifices the well-being of the larger population. In the chapter about the brain, for example, I referred to the eradication of wild-type (that is, naturally occurring) polio from the Western Hemisphere in 1991. In 2000, however, there was an outbreak of nineteen cases in the Dominican Republic. The virus causing the epidemic was isolated, and surprisingly it was more similar to the vaccine virus than the wild-type virus. Somehow, the vaccine had mutated into a form that wasn't harmless anymore. In the Dominican Republic, researchers concluded that the polio vaccine virus regained its virulence—the opposite process of attenuation—due to poor vaccine coverage. Just as the creators of the vaccine cultured the original poliovirus repeatedly until a mutation rendered it nonpathogenic, the citizens of the Dominican Republic reversed the process. They allowed a harmless virus to keep infecting unimmunized people until it acquired enough mutations to again cause paralysis. For a while, then, polio emerged from its grave until an exhaustive vaccination program placed it again in its coffin.

A related argument for public good applies to varicella vaccine. Opponents of universal varicella vaccination point out that less than 2 percent of adults today are susceptible to chickenpox. Assuming that vaccine immunity to chickenpox wanes faster than natural immunity (a contention not yet supported by any data), wouldn't vaccination create a larger pool of adults who might get chickenpox at an older age, when the disease can be more severe? The answer depends.

Suppose two elderly parents live in a large family home with twenty children, of whom sixteen are immune to varicella. Assume that one child is exposed randomly to chickenpox at school. There is an 80 percent chance that this particular child has immunity and won't spread the virus to his elderly parents when he returns home. Now suppose that only six of twenty children are immune. It's now much more likely that a child exposed at school will bring the contagion home to her parents. The probability that the elderly parents would be protected is now only 40 percent. The point is, as long as a large majority is vaccinated, diseases will very rarely spread to susceptible people. This is called "herd immunity." Mathematical models show that varicella vaccine coverage must approach 90 percent to ensure herd immunity. Anything less can be hazardous. As the American Academy of Pediatrics asserts, "[Physicians] who withhold varicella immunization from young children because of fear of creating a cohort of adults at risk for serious varicella disease may be creating a self-fulfilling prophecy." When deciding whether to get vaccinations, people make decisions for society, not just for themselves.

Returning to Patrick Powell, I encouraged his father to consider varicella vaccine for any other children in his family, since a susceptible child who gets the vaccine immediately after exposure can sometimes avoid the disease. Patrick's father asked if the painful rash he had two weeks ago was related to his son's illness. "My doctor said I had shingles," he said. He initially felt burning pain in a scythe-shaped pattern extending from his back around to his chest, and then a rash developed in this area.

In 1888, a German physician noted that children like Patrick developed chickenpox after exposure to someone with shingles. An unethical researcher later produced chickenpox in children by dubiously inoculating them with fluid from patients with shingles. Today doctors believe that after infecting the skin, the chickenpox virus invades nerves near the skin, and travels back to the spinal cord. There it lies dormant for the duration of a person's life, until waning immunity triggers its reemergence. The virus bursts out of the affected nerve, whose path is outlined on the overlying skin. The affected skin is just as contagious as that of a child with chickenpox.

Though some children develop shingles, the condition primarily affects adults. The pain, according to a usually muted medical textbook, can be "excruciating." A variety of medications is used for treatment but is often ineffective. As Patrick's father told me, "It was hell." I told him the shingles likely caused his son's chickenpox. Of note, preliminary data suggest that the vaccine also decreases the risk of shingles; the nerves likely become latently infected with the harmless vaccine virus instead of the virulent wild-type virus.

Having experienced what they now knew was a shared suffering, son and father prepared to leave. Patrick pulled on a down jacket to which I affixed a sticker he chose, which read, "Be Nice to Me. I Just Saw the Doctor." I returned to the doctor's station and picked up the next chart in line.

It's ironic that my own father, who was taking medication that weakened his immune system, called me shortly afterward to tell me he had developed shingles. This was the latest in a long succession of hardships he had braved. I desperately hoped that a curative lung transplant might happen soon, so he could stop taking the immunosuppressant drugs that likely caused the shingles. But back then I didn't anticipate the events that would transpire within a year, beginning with a phone call in the middle of one night when I was visiting him in New Jersey.

My family's phone doesn't ring at 1 A.M. with good news, and it was 1 A.M. and the phone was ringing. I knocked over a glass of water reaching for the receiver. "Your father's desaturating and going to be intubated," said the nurse in the intensive care unit. She didn't say more since she knew I am a physician. The words conveyed a basic message: my father had suddenly deteriorated and would be placed on a breathing machine.

Earlier that day my sister and I had rushed him to the emergency room, where he was found to have a collapsed lung, a complication of his underlying disease. This was relieved by the insertion of a tube into his chest, and he immediately felt better. Admitted only for observation, he was expected home in a few days. We had left the hospital only one hour earlier to sleep at home.

In my mind's eye, I went over the procedure my father likely would undergo. He'd receive some fentanyl (a form of morphine), midazolam (a form of Valium), and something called succinyl-choline, a compound with properties similar to cobra venom that paralyzes one's muscles. Thus sedated, my father would have a plas-tic tube the size of a cigar placed through his mouth and into his windpipe. Then a mechanical ventilator would breath for him. I myself had initiated this procedure many times; it was routine and complications were rare. But my hands shook slightly as I drove at high speed with my family to the hospital. "Stay within the lines," said my sister, who is also a physician.

With effort, I pushed intrusive emotions from my mind. Medical crises demand an economy of thought and feeling, a channeled use of mental resources. My father needed his son the doctor. Years ear-lier, I had offered only emotional support for him as he told me of his trouble breathing. I left the doctoring to his doctor and acted like a son. That was a mistake. One day my sister and I reviewed his medical records and found he had been grossly mismanaged. A new specialist we located made the diagnosis of idiopathic pulmonary fibrosis, a progressive scarring condition of the lungs. There is no effective treatment, and my father had become increasingly depen-dent on high-flow oxygen, which he now inhaled through a mask.

We arrived at the intensive care unit and I became increasingly analytical. Masses of monitors measured the parameters of my father's body, including arterial blood pressure, pulmonary artery pressure, capillary wedge pressure, urine output, partial pressure of inspired oxygen, and others. I read the numbers like omens. With a calculator, I figured his electrolyte balance, caloric needs, and frac-tional excretion of sodium. His blood pressure was stable on vaso-pressor medications and the oxygen saturation of his hemoglobin was stable. Satisfied his doctors were doing everything right, I returned to the small waiting area to my family. There was nothing more I could do to help him.

I sat in a chair facing my grieving mother, and noted that her image became slightly refracted by excess saline in my eyes. I explained how recovery of my father's diseased lungs could take weeks and would likely never occur. Seemingly in defiance of medical probability but actually (as I later came to respect) with its acceptance, my mother sat day after day at my father's bedside and awaited his recovery. Only then did I realize the extravagances of hope she showered upon her husband, from a reservoir of faith that I lacked. I found myself increasingly dependent on her belief and less on my medical judgment. Day after day, our family sat in a small waiting room and greeted innumerable visitors bearing gifts of homemade food and also bottled water, which I drank by the case.

After two weeks, the doctors told my mother that recovery was likely impossible, and that she should consider letting my father die. After reflecting for a few days, she told me gently that it was my father's time to pass. She had no desire to watch the process, but asked my sister and me to be present.

Alone with my father and his nurse, my sister and I watched as his intravenous catheters, cardiac leads, arterial lines, oximeter, and monitors were removed. His nurse nodded to me, and turned off his ventilator. There were no parameters to watch, only my father's still body. I couldn't stand it. My hand strayed to his and my index finger palpated his radial artery, feeling the comfort of his pulse. At the moment his heart stopped, I believe I was thinking about the last bite of food my father ever chewed. It was a hospital-made grilled cheese sandwich he had bitten into carefully and then reached out to offer to my mother, who smiled at something he said.

As the eldest child, I followed Hindu custom and helped place my father's body into the crematorium after his funeral. The following day, my sister and I picked up his ashes.

We drove past the community reservoir near our house and continued on to the Delaware River. The river was frozen, except for a small area to which we walked. As my sister chanted an ancient Jain prayer, I threw handfuls of my father's ashes into the crisp water as a breeze gently returned a few particles to my forehead and cheeks and hands, embedding the fine dust into my skin.

~ 7 ~

Gonads

ON THE NEED FOR MENTIONING
THE UNMENTIONABLE

In the middle of the night, I once treated a teenage boy who had a positive pregnancy test. "My stuff hurts," he'd told the triage nurse of the emergency room, and that's all he would say.

Jasper Davis was a seventeen-year-old high schooler from Roxbury, a predominantly African-American area of Boston. I looked at him closely, since he looked familiar. Then I remembered having seen him six months earlier in the Adolescent Clinic for a checkup. Among other things, he had wanted to discuss an unsightly bulge over his thigh. It turned out to be a bullet embedded under the skin. "Got shot," he explained.

The former Boston City Hospital attracts a colorful array of patients; a colleague remembers seeing a teen who carried two pagers, one labeled "Bitches" and the other "Bizness." The seamy side of urban life often was on display. In the pediatric emergency room, we treated sexually transmitted diseases, trauma from gang violence, and rape. The latter complaint is frequent enough that emergency rooms stock blue-lettered boxes called "rape kits," with a step-by-step pamphlet instructing doctors on how to collect forensic evidence from children using a variety of swabs.

Despite his street-tough veneer, Jasper was an engaging individual. He wanted to graduate from high school and attend a community college. At his previous visit, we spent time reviewing safe sex practices. Like most adolescents, he welcomed such discussions with a doctor. In one Boston study, 80 percent of high school students wanted to hear about safe sex from their pediatricians, but only half felt comfortable initiating such a discussion. Additionally, 85 percent of parents wanted their children to get information on safe sex. This reflects acceptance of a powerful fact: nationwide, about 50 percent of high school students have had sexual intercourse, half of them before reaching sixteen years of age and a third before thirteen years of age. African-American adolescents like Jasper are the most sexually active ethnic group; three-quarters report having had intercourse at least once. Often, students not having intercourse participate in other sexual activities. In Los Angeles, one-third of students describing themselves as virgins had engaged in masturbation with an opposite sex partner, and 10 percent had performed oral sex.

At our first visit, Jasper had shuffled into the exam room, hiked up his oversized jeans, and draped himself over a chair. A small tattoo on his arm read "Never." He cocked his head back, and his expression would have indicated surprise if his eyes hadn't remained hooded. He exuded boredom. Surprisingly, it was easy to get him to talk using a common technique. To help clinicians gain a window into an adolescent's world, two pediatricians at the Children's Hospital of Los Angeles created a structured interviewing method called

Getting into Adolescents' HEADSS to uncover high-risk behaviors. The letters stand respectively for Home, Education/Employment, Activities, Drugs, Sexuality, and Suicide/Depression.

In America, viruses and bacteria are not the main killers of adolescents. The major causes of mortality are car accidents (usually involving alcohol or drugs), suicide, and homicide. Additionally, school failure, teen pregnancy, and sexually transmitted diseases are epidemic. One in ten sexually active female teens carries chlamydia, a common venereal disease, and about a third of teenagers have ridden in a car with an intoxicated driver. One key principle of adolescent medicine is that warning signs precede adverse outcomes, and an astute pediatrician can identify these signs early and intervene. Because no self-respecting adolescent immediately volunteers details of his or her sexual and drug habits, a doctor first needs to create rapport. That's where the HEADSS interview comes in.

Beginning with his home life, I asked Jasper, "How many brothers and sisters do you have? How do you get along?" He explained he was the oldest of four children, all sharing a single bedroom in a high-rise project tower. He and his brother Tyrone collected baseball cards and comic books, which didn't interest his sisters. "We all get along pretty well," he said. "How about your parents?" I continued.

Jasper's father had left his mother some time ago. "My momma keeps me on track," Jasper said, grinning. Speaking about families is a nonthreatening way to initiate a discussion with adolescents. Despite teens' need for individuation, families are still the center of their lives and a fruitful topic of conversation. From there, we talked about Jasper's friends and his school performance. His favorite subjects were English and gym class. "Are you failing any classes?" I asked. "Yeah, math. But my mom got me a tutor," he replied. He denied any suspensions. "What kinds of things do you and your friends do outside of school?" I asked. He mentioned basketball, skateboarding, and hanging out at a local dance club.

Progressively, we explored Jasper's high-risk behaviors, using his friends as a conversational entrée. Yeah, he admitted, his friends smoked marijuana frequently and used cocaine occasionally. I asked, "It's very common to experiment with drugs. Have you also tried them?" Like many teens given permission to disclose drug use, Jasper readily admitted that he had. But distinguishing casual experimentation from abuse can be tricky; for example, the majority of high schoolers have used alcohol and marijuana at least once, and most ultimately lead healthy lives. Several screening tests exist to identify high-risk youth. Perhaps the best known is the C.A.G.E. questionnaire, developed in 1974 to identify alcohol dependence by asking four questions: whether a patient feels she must *cut down* on drinking, feels *annoyed* by comments about her drinking, ever experiences *guilt* about drinking, or needs an alcohol-containing *eye-opener* early in the day. Any person answering two or more affirmatives is at risk of unhealthy alcohol use and needs further assessment. I asked Jasper a variation of these questions for illicit drug use, and concluded his marijuana use was likely recreational.

We moved on and I said, "Developing close relationships is a part of maturing, and so is physical intimacy. When do you think that people are ready for sex?" Looking at the floor and sliding his feet around, Jasper said, "I don't know. Whenever they are." It's funny how some doctors ask whether someone is "sexually active," since the terminology is confusing. I'm much more direct, and asked Jasper, "About how long ago was the last time you had sex?" Though some adolescents issue indignant denials, many are open about their behavior. "Last month," said Jasper. I pressed on, "Are your preferred partners men, women, or both?" Jasper looked at me incredulously and exclaimed, "Hey, I'm no fag." Though a charged question, it's worth asking. One to 2 percent of high schoolers view themselves as mostly or completely homosexual, and fully 10 percent are unsure.

Like about half of teens, Jasper hadn't used a condom during his last intercourse. He somewhat sheepishly admitted that his last girlfriend was a few weeks pregnant. We spent about ten minutes talking about proper condom use. Fewer than one in ten males has ever received medical instruction on proper condom use, including correct placement and need for withdrawal shortly after ejaculation. Likely due to incorrect use, a quarter of sexually active males report that their condom broke during intercourse over the past year. I asked Jasper to carry one at all times; one study showed that teens with available condoms are three times more likely to use them consistently. Because scaring teens about AIDS hasn't been shown to improve condom use, I simply tried to get Jasper to understand that safe sex is a mutual responsibility between partners.

After completing the HEADSS interview, I performed a routine physical, including a scoliosis check and cardiac exam. While examining Jasper's genitals, I showed him how to palpate his testicle and feel the comma-shaped organ at its apex called the epididymis. "You should do this every month while taking a shower, and let your doctor know if you ever feel a hard bump," I said. I gave him a little plastic hanger for his showerhead that pictured the procedure. I also wrote a referral to a surgeon to extract the bullet from his body. "I was just standing there, and I got shot," Jasper explained, and I didn't press him for details. We shook hands and he left. I didn't think we'd meet again.

But we did, six months later, at three in the morning the night his "stuff hurt." He didn't seem surprised to see me.

"Remember that thing about examining my balls?" Jasper said. "I did that tonight 'cause I couldn't sleep and it feels kind of hard down there." I don't know what possessed the boy to examine his testicles at three in the morning, and didn't ask, although I suspected the answer would be lively. He continued, "I didn't want to tell the nurse. You see what I'm saying. It's my stuff."

In an exam room, Jasper removed his jeans and pulled down his boxers. His sexual development was normal for his age. The first sign of puberty in boys is an increase in testicular size. At the previous visit, I'd sized one of his testicles with my right hand, and with the left held a rosary-like string of increasingly larger yellow plastic balls called a goniometer, which I rotated until finding a ball approximating the size of Jasper's testicle. I glanced at the size indicated by the goniometer: about fifteen cubic centimeters, which was normal for late adolescence. His pubic hair covered the base of the penis and spread slightly to his thighs, which was also normal.

An acutely painful scrotum is a medical emergency. The most common cause in young children is that the testicle twists around, tangling the blood vessels that supply it. If left untreated for over six hours, the affected testicle asphyxiates and dies. In older boys like Jasper, the most common cause of scrotal pain is infection of the epididymis, which is usually sexually acquired. However, Jasper's mild pain wasn't typical for these conditions, since those kids usually writhe in agony.

I examined Jasper carefully. As reported, his left testicle had a rock-hard area the size of a blueberry. His penis appeared normal, with no discharge to suggest an active gonorrheal or chlamydial infection. He pulled up his boxers and I turned to his belly, which appeared normal. When listening to his heart, though, I noticed something fairly odd. Jasper was growing breasts.

During early puberty, two-thirds of boys experience a small degree of breast growth, a condition called gynecomastia. Over the years, I've probably seen at least a dozen panicked teenage boys in the clinic with the condition only to reassure them that it is normal and usually goes away by itself. Rarely, there are other explanations. In 1979, an epidemic of breast development among Italian schoolboys may have been caused by estrogen-contaminated meat. In Baltimore, I'd once seen a young male prostitute who intentionally took estrogens to grow breasts to please his clientele. In other boys, the growth may be caused by certain antifungal medications or excessive marijuana smoking. (The latter effect is an ideal negative reinforcer for a boy's illicit drug use. Marijuana, by the way, doesn't enhance breast growth in girls.) Jasper had had no breast growth at his last visit, and new enlargement this late in puberty was concerning.

"We'll need to draw some blood," I said to him. I drew a teaspoon's worth from his arm, labeled it, and sent it to the laboratory. While waiting for results, I ordered an ultrasound of his scrotum to better define the mass. I wrote out a form indicating my concern, handed it to Jasper, and pointed the way to radiology. He swaggered off. After fifteen minutes, I punched up his blood test on the computer. I'd sent a pregnancy test—and it was positive.

A pregnancy test measures human chorionic gonadotropin, or HCG, made by the placenta in a gestating woman. The positive test meant Jasper too had HCG, a hormone whose presence can cause gynecomastia. He certainly couldn't be carrying a child, so where was it coming from? The testicle mass must have had something to do with it. I walked over to radiology and found Jasper. The radiologist said, "It's probably what you think." I nodded and led Jasper back to the exam room, where we sat down. I told Jasper what his problem was.

Several thousand American men every year develop Jasper's disease, which was testicular cancer. It is the most common tumor in males between fifteen and thirty-four years of age. The tumor is aggressive and typically grows with surprising rapidity, doubling in size every three weeks or so. Medical students around the country have seen slides of one African villager with the cancer who trekked scores of miles to see a surgeon, all the while carting along his watermelon-sized testicle in a wheelbarrow. In developed countries, though, testicular cancer has become eminently treatable. In the 1960s, 40 percent of patients with the problem died; today, only 5 percent succumb to it.

Though critical in puberty, the testicle does precious little immediately after a child's birth, lulled by a lack of activating hormones from the brain. Then sometime around ten years of age, the brain decides—for reasons no one fully understands—to start puberty. The process begins at nighttime: every hour or so, the pituitary spurts messenger molecules called follicle-stimulating hormone and lutenizing hormone into the blood. This pulsatile activity arouses the testes from their slumber like an insistent knocking at the door. In response, the testes expand to meet their new manufacturing responsibilities: making sperm and releasing testosterone into the blood. Puberty begins as the penis enlarges, the voice changes, pubic and underarm hair appear, and other changes occur. In girls, the ovaries respond instead of the testes, and make estrogens that ultimately cause breast enlargement and menstruation.

Like the ovary, the testicle is an endocrine gland, meaning that it controls distant areas of the body via hormones. When affected by cancer, endocrine cells can undergo a bizarre transformation and suddenly acquire the ability to release hormones they were never intended to make. It's as if the cells become psychic; they somehow channel the powers of other organs, fetal cells, or, occasionally, cells of the opposite sex. For example, certain liver tumors make alphafetoprotein (normally made by a placenta), some lung cancers make antidiuretic hormone (whose synthesis is usually reserved for the brain), and, as in Jasper's case, many testicular tumors make the female hormone HCG.

Chaos frequently results. In women, HCG performs a key role during pregnancy, but it has no place in a young man's body. Because of the HCG, Jasper developed breasts and even had some symptoms (elicited by specific questioning) that could be construed as morning sickness. On the bright side, the HCG could also be used as a tool to help Jasper. When production of HCG is interrupted—for example, by surgery or chemotherapy of the cancer—the body clears the hormone within a week. After treatment was begun, a simple blood test could then tell if Jasper was cured. No HCG would mean no tumor.

I broke the bad news to Jasper and spoke uninterrupted for ten minutes. He sighed and looked bored, an expression he must have learned long ago to hide his feelings. "So what are they gonna do?" he said. I answered, "You need surgery to remove your left testicle. Then, depending on whether the tumor has spread, you may need radiation or chemotherapy. Then you'll need checkups every few months, maybe for years. It's possible you might become sterile, so you may need to bank your sperm, too. But your surgeon will tell you all about that." He nodded, put his hands in his pockets, and looked away. I got up and paged the urologist on call. A tired-sounding voice answered on the phone, and I heard the rustle of bedsheets. The resident said, "Just have him come to the clinic in the morning, nine o'clock. We'll get him booked then." I told Jasper the plan.

"Sounds good," he intoned. "Am I all set to go, then?" I prepared his discharge paperwork and handed him a slip for his morning appointment with the urologist. As before, we shook hands and he left.

After a minute, someone tapped me on the shoulder at the nurse's station. It was Jasper, who asked, "You know, with this problem I got, does that mean I can't have sex tonight?" Taken aback, I advised against it until he saw the urologist. Then I remembered something from our previous meeting.

"Hey, what happened to your girlfriend, the one who was pregnant?" I asked. "Her?" he said. "Oh, yeah. She got an abortion."

Jasper's comment reminded me of another night a few years earlier, when I performed my first and only abortion. Having done an abor-

tion is something that fills me with neither pride nor embarrassment, but I do look back with some sorrow. I'll explain why briefly.

Teen pregnancy is not a new problem. In his play *The Winter's
Tale*, Shakespeare lamented, "I wish there were no age between ten
and twenty-three, or that youth would sleep out the rest; for there is
nothing in the between but getting wenches with child." Today,
most girls begin menstruating between eleven and thirteen years of
age. Given their early debut of sexual intercourse and generally poor
utilization of contraception, about *one in ten* American girls
between the ages of fifteen and nineteen gets pregnant every year,
and 90 percent of these are unintended. Like fifteen-year-old
Lakeesha Davis, slightly over a third of these pregnant teens end up
getting abortions.

A withdrawn girl accompanied by her mother, Lakeesha wore
her hair neatly braided in cornrows and dressed in loose-fitting
jeans and a leather jacket. (At the place where I did my gynecology
rotation as a medical student, patients could secure abortions by
coming to the emergency room.) Lakeesha took a seat in an exam
room and answered my questions in a monotone. She had been
having sex for about a year, and generally relied on condoms for
contraception. Her last period occurred ten weeks ago. She had
never had an abortion. She was nervous, but her mother said she'd
accompany her through the procedure.

Lakeesha's baby was now the length of a golf ball. About eight
weeks ago, Lakeesha had sexual intercourse with her boyfriend,
when she said the "condom broke." Millions of sperm from her
partner traveled through her vagina and entered her uterus, then
made their way to her fallopian tubes. In previous decades, the
process of fertilization was described as "warrior sperm" seeking
"damsel-in-distress eggs" until anthropologist Emily Martin objected
that such analogies are sexist. Martin pointed out that the female
menstrual cycle was described by textbooks as involving "denuding,"

"dying," and expulsion of "debris," while sperm production was called "amazing," especially with its "sheer magnitude of producing millions of sperm a day." One quaint source she cited explained how the egg "drifts" and is passively "swept" into the fallopian tubes, where "streamlined" sperm with "strong" tails then "activate" gestation by "penetrating" the egg.

In any event, when a single sperm successfully docked, the egg instantly created an electrostatic field around itself to keep out other sperm. Conception had occurred. Over the next four days, the fertilized egg migrated down the fallopian tubes into the uterus, and divided into a ball made of about thirty-two cells. Then, around the fifth day, the ball hatched out of the egg's protective covering called the zona pellucida and attached to Lakeesha's uterus. A placenta developed at that site and released HCG into the blood. Like Jasper, Lakeesha developed a positive pregnancy test.

"Did you consider a morning-after pill when you found out the condom broke?" I asked Lakeesha. She looked at me blankly. Like almost 85 percent of students who get abortions, Lakeesha hadn't heard of this method, which has been available in the United States for over twenty-five years and is about 75 percent effective. The regimen is exceedingly simple: within three days of unprotected intercourse, two pills of Ovral, a type of birth control pill, are taken twice. In England alone, it has been used four million times to prevent pregnancy. Though in 1996 the World Health Organization added the medication to its "essential drugs list," few American pediatricians mention its existence to adolescents during routine checkups. Perhaps it's underutilized because it's often confused with abortion; however, the pill doesn't actually terminate a pregnancy—it prevents it. The pill either prevents conception in the first place by delaying ovulation or changes the uterine lining to prevent implantation.

After I explained the 1 percent risk of complication associated with abortions, Lakeesha fixed me squarely with her gaze and said evenly, "I want an abortion." Consent papers were signed, routine blood tests ordered, and an operating room readied. After an hour, the supervising resident named Alicia Jones and I went upstairs to prepare for the procedure. After changing into pale green scrubs, we each stood in front of large steel sinks and systematically rubbed a plastic brush impregnated with antibacterial soap over our forearms, twenty-five times in each of a dozen planes. Holding our arms upward, we kicked open the door to the operating room where the circulating nurses efficiently draped us in sterile blue gowns. Lastly, I thrust my hands into latex gloves held by the nurse.

Laskeesha lay on her back, sedated with a narcotic. The anesthesiologist had also injected a medication into the spinal canal that would last several hours. Lakeesha's torso and legs were numb. Two nurses placed Lakeesha's legs apart in elevated stirrups so her pelvis was exposed. Alicia nodded, and I sat on a stool between the stirrups, facing Lakeesha. To my right, Alicia laid a gleaming array of surgical instruments on a metal table.

"First," said Alicia, "you need to dilate the cervix. Use this." She handed me an oblong metal rod and guided my hand so we placed the instrument into Lakeesha's vagina and advanced the tip five inches to the cervix, the entrance to the uterus. "Push it through," Alicia continued. I did and felt a slight give. I pulled out the rod, and Alicia handed me a thicker one, and instructed me to insert it. "We'll keep doing this with larger instruments until the cervix is opened enough to insert the vacuum."

My eyes must have betrayed me. "You know," said Alicia stiffly, "that it's easy to pay lip service to a woman's right to choose. Are you ready to put your money where your mouth is?" I recalled a scene from John Irving's *The Cider House Rules,* where the protagonist, a budding gynecologist named Homer Wells, refuses to perform an abortion on a girl, despite being the only trained surgeon around. The girl ends up getting a botched procedure from an untrained practitioner. The amateur abortionist dumps the girl on

Homer's doorstep with her panties pinned to her blouse and a note unceremoniously admonishing Homer, "Shit or get off the pot." Alicia was basically saying the same thing to me.

I nodded. A shaft of flesh ten weeks earlier had deposited the seed of a baby's life. Now, bright ones of metal would take it away. When the dilation was completed, Alicia inserted her hand into Lakeesha's vagina and felt her cervix, now open a few centimeters. "It's ready," she pronounced. "Insert the vacuum."

We placed a clear plastic tube through the cervix and flipped a switch. With a sucking noise, the tube filled with reddish tissue extracted from Laskeesha's uterus. I moved the tube back and forth through the uterus until the flow stopped, then removed it from Lakeesha's body. The pulpy extract collected in a strainerlike device, and Alicia and I poured its contents onto a sterile dish. "Did you get it?" Alicia asked me. With forceps, I picked through the tissue, which looked like clots of blood. Then I saw it: a pale, short piece of debris as wide as a matchstick. At the tip, I recognized small protrusions that were—without any doubt—five small fingers. I've never forgotten the sight. As a child, I once behaved so badly that my mother hauled off and slapped me across the face as hard as she could. For several days my cheeks had shown the imprint of her fingers, a reminder of my transgression. Almost twenty years later, those fingers of Lakeesha's never-to-be-born child left another, even more persistent imprint on me. I had intentionally killed an unborn child.

What I had just done occurs legally twenty-six million times a year in the world and twenty million times a year illegally. Women who get abortions assume great risk if they do so in areas where abortion is prohibited. From complications of illegal abortions, 78,000 women die preventable deaths every year, a number of people more than twenty-five times greater than those killed in the World Trade Center attacks of September 11. Making abortion illegal doesn't appear to stop a woman from getting one; it forces her to hire an amateur instead of a professional.

Though abortion is relatively inaccessible to many Americans, the United States has one of the highest abortion rates among developed countries. This is remarkable because 86 percent of counties have no abortion providers or facilities. When a scarce provider is found, the poor find that Medicaid won't pay for an abortion. In 1991, the Supreme Court ruled in *Rust v. Sullivan* that providers at health facilities that accept federal funds couldn't even *mention* the existence of abortion, and upheld the so-called abortion gag rule. (Bill Clinton reversed this gag rule, which was promptly reinstated by George W. Bush on the anniversary of *Roe v. Wade*, and expanded to cover any overseas health organizations that receive U.S. funds.) Although mifepristone, which is more notoriously known as the abortion pill RU-486, was approved over a decade ago in France and caused no increase in that country's abortion rates (the same trend was seen in Sweden and England following mifepristone's approval), political pressure prevented its approval in the United States for over a decade. American policy makers consistently operate with the mistaken belief that making an abortion harder to get makes getting one less likely. It doesn't. For example, the percentages of American teens that abort are 33, 200, and 500 higher than their respective counterparts in Canada, France, and the Netherlands, where abortions are far easier to obtain.

After snapping off our gloves and sterile gowns, we scrubbed out of the operating room. I told Alicia the procedure was unpleasant to perform. She wasn't moved. She lectured, "Look, nobody likes doing them. If we don't do them, the patient will find somebody else who will and maybe screw it up. And anyway, you didn't do anything you didn't want to do."

Somewhat chastised, I went to see Lakeesha for her postoperative examination. Her anesthesia had likely worn off and she'd probably start having cramps. I wrote an order for some pain medication. "How do you feel?" I asked. With pursed lips, she shook her head and said nothing. She looked distraught, and though I sat down and waited for her to speak, I might as well have been a million miles away. Filling time, I discussed routine postoperative care and made an appointment for her to return to the clinic in a few days. Leaving the room, I realized that she hadn't said anything after signing the form authorizing her abortion. In the hall I passed Lakeesha's mother, who acknowledged me with a polite nod and moved along.

Though they often describe their primary motivation as a need to help others, physicians operate with the hidden hubris that they play an integral role in other people's lives. When we suture lacerations, treat ear infections, find vitamin deficiencies, or deliver babies, we feel the modest thrill of being needed. This feeling is the critical positive reinforcer in our profession: why else would we tolerate a brutal training process, an exorbitantly expensive education, and prolonged deferral of normal sleeping hours if it were not to feel important to somebody every now and then? In part, I felt deflated after participating in Lakeesha's abortion because I realized I was only a bit player—a faceless technician—in a complex emotional and physical drama for her. Realizing that medical care is really about the patient and not the doctor is an obvious and necessary conclusion, but nevertheless stinging to a young physician.

But that's not why I look back on that night with sorrow. That emotion arises from the central feature of the abortion: it had been preventable. American teens don't get more abortions because they have more sex than other nations' children, because they're less prone to miscarry, or because they're more likely to abort when pregnant. We have more abortions because adolescents like Lakeesha simply don't learn enough about birth control and don't use it. Because they get pregnant more often, Americans have a half-million more abortions every year than if they got pregnant at rates more in line with certain European countries.

Those looking for a quick explanation for this phenomenon blame the media. One study found that in fifty hours of daytime soap operas, there were one hundred and fifty-six acts of intercourse, but only five references to contraception. Today, the 8:00 to 9:00 P.M. "family hour" of television contains an average of eight sexual incidents, a fourfold increase from 1976. The average teen watches seventeen hours of television weekly, and typically is exposed to 14,000 sexual references per year of which only 1 percent deal with sexually transmitted diseases, pregnancy, or contraception. By and large, television portrays sex the same way it depicts an anvil's falling on a cartoon coyote: as an act without serious consequence.

In an age with scores of contraceptive options, including daily pills, an every-three-month injection to prevent ovulation, and condoms with effective anti-infection coatings, one would think school would be an ideal venue for their discussion. However, one-third of schools have no sex education at all. Among those schools that do have a sexuality curriculum, a third teach abstinence only (which has never decreased sexual behaviors), with contraceptive information either prohibited or limited to describing lack of efficacy. Thus teens largely learn about sex from either the media or one another. One could argue that schools must mention what has too long been unmentionable. Otherwise, among other things, we're condemning a population roughly the size of Washington, D.C., every year to the same fate as Lakeesha's never-born child.

Another matter involving the pediatric reproductive system that inspires debate almost as vigorous as that surrounding abortion is the circumcision of newborn boys. Some years ago at the Brigham and Women's Hospital, I was called for a consultation to see a young professional couple named Raskin who was about to have a baby. They wanted to know the arguments for and against the practice. At the time, they didn't suspect what would soon be discovered about their baby's genitals.

Thought to have originated over six thousand years ago as depicted on the ancient tomb of Ankh-Mahor near Cairo, circumcision is likely the world's oldest operative procedure. The practice transcends diverse cultural boundaries, practiced by Jews, Muslims, certain Africans, Australian aborigines, and other groups. Though circumcision had historically been a cultural practice, P. C. Remondino in 1891 began attributing sundry health advantages to circumcision, claiming its therapeutic role in gout, asthma, alcohol dependence, seizures, and other conditions. Few physicians questioned Remondino rigorously, and the practice became common in the United States in the early twentieth century.

Previously, I had once assisted in a circumcision with an obstetrician, the doctor who does the procedure in most hospitals. We had taken a newborn boy, Evan Schneider, to the procedure room and strapped him naked to a contraption much like a car seat, which held the infant's legs spread-eagled. Using a syringe filled with lidocaine (a local anesthetic like Novocain), I visualized the base of Evan's penis as a clock, and injected a small amount at ten o'clock and two o'clock to temporarily deaden the penis. Though this seems obviously humane, most infants until recently received no pain control during circumcision, a practice stemming from a belief that babies can't localize, feel, or remember pain. However, they clearly cry, have increased blood pressure, and release copious amounts of stress hormones like cortisol into the bloodstream when a scalpel cuts the penis. In 1997, a team of Canadian researchers led by Gideon Koren found that an anesthetic cream applied to the penis reduced stress in babies undergoing circumcision, a finding deemed so revolutionary that no less an authority than the *New England Journal of Medicine* featured the article prominently to educate the medical community that, yes, babies in fact can feel pain.

Evan slowly calmed down, and we prepared our instruments. The human penis begins development at one to two months of gestation, and the foreskin that covers the penile head starts forming a month later. Initially, the foreskin adheres to the penile head as avidly as the skin on an apple. Over time, in a process not complete in some boys until after five years of age, the foreskin gradually separates from the penis, ultimately forming a retractable sleeve.

Because Evan's foreskin hadn't yet separated completely, I used a blunt probe to peel it back from the penis, as if shucking an ear of corn. The obstetrician handed me a bell-shaped plunger called a Gomco clamp, which I placed over the penile head. In final preparation, the foreskin was pulled over the bell. Using a scalpel, I then cut the foreskin circumferentially around the base of the bell, until it came off in one segment like a section of calamari. We waited a few seconds for the bleeding to stop, and the procedure was over. It had taken only ninety seconds. We soon returned Evan to his parents.

Back at the Brigham, I walked to the labor and delivery wing and met James and Emily Raskin. Lawyers in their early thirties, they hadn't yet decided whether to circumcise their child, whose prenatal sonogram had suggested male sex. "Could you," asked James, a tallish blond man with round-frame spectacles, "give the arguments for and against it?"

Circumcision had recently fallen into disfavor among Americans; today only 64 percent of boys are circumcised, compared to 80 percent in 1980. Internationally, this trend had been even more pronounced; boys in England, China, Scandinavia, and India are circumcised at rates comfortably lower than 10 percent. In large part, this decline began in 1949 when Britain's national health care system failed to find compelling evidence to support routine circumcision. In the early 1970s, Australian and Canadian pediatric health organizations came to the same conclusion, followed by the American Academy of Pediatrics in 1975. Circumcision, it seemed, was doomed as a medically indicated procedure.

Recently the tide, at least in the United States, seemed to turn in favor of circumcision as new research became available. Today, we know that circumcised infants are roughly ten times less likely to develop urinary tract infections (one in one thousand versus one in one hundred), about twenty-two times less likely to get penile cancer, and three times less likely to develop certain sexually transmitted diseases, such as HIV, as they age. This must, of course, be balanced against a 1 percent risk of complications (usually minor bleeding) from circumcision. Given this data, the American Academy of Pediatrics in 1989 proclaimed that circumcision "has potential medical benefits and advantages," but stopped short of recommending universal circumcision, instead opining that since it "is not essential to the child's well-being, parents should determine what is in the best interest of the child." Researcher Thomas Wiswell, speaking for a group of avowed foes of the AAP's position, castigated this neutral position as cowardly, and accused the AAP of "narrow, biased, and inadequate data analysis." Among other data, Wiswell cited evidence that universal male circumcision could annually save 76,000 African men from AIDS, 18,000 American infants from urinary tract infections, and 1,200 American men from invasive penile cancer.

I outlined this information for the Raskins, who listened quietly. "The bottom line," I concluded, "is that there is no consensus. It's your decision." Emily looked at James and nodded knowingly, then thanked me for my time. Since Emily was having a planned cesarean section, I'd be present at the delivery per routine to resuscitate the newborn if needed. "See you soon," I said, and left.

The arguments surrounding male circumcision strike me as largely polemical and only incidentally based on evidence (witness any exchange of letters on the subject in scientific journals). In contrast, "circumcision" of young girls as practiced in Africa inspires condemnation from many parties, and rightly so. Nahid Toubia, a surgeon with extensive experience in Sudan, explains that "circumcision" is really a misleading term for what 5 to 99 percent of girls in various African societies undergo typically between the ages of four and ten years with no anesthesia. In Type I and II procedures, the clitoris and part of the labia minora are cut off, and the raw remaining surfaces are closed with thorns or stitches of catgut. In anatomic terms, this is analogous to removal of the entire male penis, and not just the foreskin. In more radical Type III and IV cases, termed infibulations, the entire labia minora, clitoris, and portions of the labia majora are excised, leaving only a small opening for passage of urine and menstrual blood. About one hundred million women in the world have had these procedures performed, which are illegal in most modern societies and condemned by the World Health Organization. Even in the United States, though, desire for the procedure exists: I recently saw an Ethiopian refugee in a Boston clinic who asked me where her daughter could get it done.

It was evening, so I walked from the labor and delivery floor to the cafeteria and bought a turkey and Swiss cheese sandwich on rye bread. I got the same thing whenever on call. Residency was something like boot camp, and I automatically adapted a militaristic eating style. I sat with a colleague and we ate our rations. Halfway through the meal, my friend's pager went off and he excused himself after stuffing half a sandwich into his mouth. My own pager chirped shortly afterward, ending a typical dinner.

Emily Raskin was being taken into the operating room for her C-section, so I changed into scrubs and unpacked my tackle box. The procedure went smoothly, and I shot the breeze with the circulating nurse while waiting for the baby. "Water's broken," I heard, meaning that the uterus had been opened. From below my field of view came vigorous cries, and James said to Emily, "He's here!"

The obstetrician looked up at James and, while removing the baby, called out, "Congratulations. You have a beautiful . . ." A pause ensued as the doctor saw the child's genitals, and concluded, "child."

The scrub nurse handed the infant to me, and I brought the child over to the warmer and dried the writhing body with clean towels. I systematically assessed the baby's lungs and heartbeat, which were fine. The baby's color rapidly went from blue to a healthy rosy shade. But there was an immediate problem: I couldn't tell if the baby was a boy or a girl. At the baby's pelvis there was a one-centimeter-long appendage that looked like a penis. However, at the base, in place of a scrotum containing testicles, there instead was a length-wise opening bordered by swollen tissue resembling labia majora. The child possessed parts of both sexes, and I couldn't assign a male or female gender. The child had what pediatricians call ambiguous genitalia.

"Your child has a problem with the genitals," I said to James, after walking over. "It's unclear whether you have a boy or girl, and we'll need to do some tests to investigate." I showed the problem to James, wrapped the child in clean linens, and handed the newborn over. James silently kissed the baby's forehead and looked worried. Still sedated, Emily slept. Her husband would have to break the news when she woke. I explained the evaluation to James and tried to offer some reassurance. Then he handed his baby back to me, and I took the child to the NICU to determine what happened to the gonads during their development, which began about eight months ago.

We all have an inborn tendency to develop into females. That is, a developing human's gonads at one to two months of gestation become ovaries when left alone. Internal pouches called mullerian ducts gradually become the fallopian tubes, uterus, and upper vagina, and externally the labia minora and majora appear; this is the default pathway of our bodies.

It is the presence of a single piece of DNA called the SRY gene—the key portion of the Y-chromosome—that turns males into males. By a process not fully understood, the SRY gene makes the month-old gonads inside the fetus's abdomen into testicles. But that isn't what ultimately makes one into a male. A remarkable cascade ensues involving human chorionic gonadotropin (HCG), the hormone detected by pregnancy tests. From the mother's placenta, HCG percolates into fetal bloodstream and induces the testes to make testosterone. (HCG has no clear effect on ovaries.) Testosterone then alters the natural tendency of the genitals to become female. Not only are we all preprogrammed to become female, but those of us who do become male are only so because our mothers' bodies decreed it.

A fetus's transformation from femaleness to maleness occurs in three parts. First, the testicles make a substance called antimullerian hormone, or AMH, that makes the mullerian ducts wither away. Thus, internal female genitals cannot develop. Second, testosterone causes other pouches, called wolffian ducts, to become the vas deferens, epididymis, and seminal vesicles, which eventually connect the testicles to the penis. As gestation proceeds, these organs and the testes move out of the abdomen and into the scrotum. Lastly, the skin of the fetus's developing genitals (which contain an enzyme called 5-alpha reductase, which has significance for a Dominican Republic culture that I will discuss) converts testosterone into dihydrotestosterone, or DHT. DHT molds the skin of the pelvis into a penis and scrotum instead of a clitoris and labia, respectively, giving the child the external appearance of a boy. In summary, the hormones AMH, testosterone, and DHT make Y-chromosome-carrying fetuses look like boys on the inside and outside.

A child with ambiguous genitals almost always has one of two conditions. There could be female genes (two X-chromosomes) but an inappropriate, hidden source of male hormones like AMH, testosterone, or DHT. This child would have ovaries, but have some male-appearing genitals. Alternatively, there could be male genes (one X-chromosome and one Y-chromosome), but some problem in making or responding to male hormones. In this situation, the child would have testes (sometimes hidden in the abdomen), but also have some female-appearing genitals.

In the NICU, James and Emily Raskin's baby was placed in an open bassinet. Usually, the cribs of NICU entrants have blue or pink cards with the child's name. Our new patient got a white one. Because English has no gender-neutral pronoun for people (the word "it" seems inappropriate), we referred to our charge repeatedly as "the baby." The attending neonatologist named Edward Stringer and I conferred.

A rotund man with an exuberant sense of humor, Edward was always in motion, tapping his fingers, humming melodies, or bouncing in his chair. When writing with his right hand, his left unconsciously mirrored the motions. Between discussions about patients one day, he once purchased a potato-powered clock using a lab result terminal connected to the Internet. But his exterior hid a man of singular intelligence, for he was the director of the NICU and an accomplished researcher.

Edward recommended that we first determine what the baby's chromosomes were. We drew a whiff of blood and sent it to the lab immediately, but an answer would take forty-eight hours. Then he called a radiologist to delineate the baby's internal anatomy. Finally, we drew some more blood to measure various hormone levels. "For now," he said, "we wait." He walked away, tapping various bassinets in his path.

I looked down at our patient, who stirred briefly before turning to one side and falling asleep. I wondered if the child was dreaming. The workings of infants' brains are enigmatic, especially regarding their development of sexual identity. In 1967, a family practitioner performed a negligent circumcision on a healthy newborn boy, and destroyed the penis. Seen by Dr. John Money, a noted sexologist from Johns Hopkins, the boy's parents were advised to complete a sex-change operation on the child, hide his birth sex from him, and raise him as a girl. Money subscribed to the notion that sexual identity is socially constructed, and thus malleable. But, as described by reporter John Colapinto in his book *As Nature Made Him*, the child grew up with great sexual frustration and ambivalence, and after growing up as a teen girl decided to live as an adult man. In contrast to Money's beliefs, the child's gender identity seemed fixed very early, likely by hereditary factors.

In this regard, the transformation of *guevedoces* from the southwestern part of the Dominican Republic is especially instructive. Lacking normal 5-alpha-reductase in their developing genitals because of a genetic defect, certain male fetuses are unable to convert testosterone into DHT. These infants have normal AMH and testosterone, but lack DHT. Consequently, these newborns have testes and numerous male structures that remain in the abdomen, but have exterior genitals that appear female. Everything about them is male except for their external genitals. They are initially reared as females, since that's what they look like.

But around puberty, the pituitary gland activates the testes to make large amounts of testosterone. Though DHT is still absent, testosterone in these large quantities can mimic the effects of DHT. Suddenly, in early puberty, these individuals begin *growing a penis*. (*Guevedoces* literally means "penis at twelve years.") They develop a deepened voice, chest hair, and other signs of maleness. They subsequently live as males, identify themselves as males, and may report that they always felt like males trapped in female bodies. This further supports the lessons of the Hopkins case: a person's gender identity may be determined very early in development by testosterone.

In the NICU, the Raskin baby did well after admission, having no obvious problems other than the ambiguous genitals. Later in the day, I held the child for a while sitting in a rocking chair and fed the child an ounce of formula. According to the nurse, the baby cried and slept like any other newborn. The only clue to the baby's problem was the parade of surgeons, endocrinologists, radiologists, and neonatologists who intermittently came to examine the baby's genitals.

The radiologist was the first to present helpful information. The sonogram showed that the child internally had a uterus and vagina. The mullerian ducts had not withered, which meant that no AMH was ever made. It was therefore likely that the child didn't have testicles (which would have made AMH) but ovaries. In addition, there did not appear to be any obvious male structures other than the small appendage resembling a penis.

It was likely that the child was a genetic female, meaning she had two X-chromosomes. Why, then, did the baby have a partial penis? We found out very shortly, when the lab called with the results of a blood test.

The answer begins with a complex, commonly known molecule that is the building block of our sex hormones. Biochemist Joseph Goldstein calls it "the most highly decorated small molecule in biology," since thirteen Nobel Prizes have been awarded for its study. Among other functions, various hormones derived from it shape our genitals, maintain our blood pressure, build up our muscles, and help fight infection. Primarily made by the liver, the molecule begins with tiny pieces of sugar that are joined, twisted, and oxidized in a dizzying series to make an end product faintly resembling the interlinked Olympic rings. This molecule is cholesterol.

Like crude oil, cholesterol is transported from the site of its production, the liver, by tankers called chylomicrons to refineries throughout the body. In the testes, for example, cholesterol brought by chylomicrons is converted into testosterone, in the ovaries it's made into estrogen, and in the kidneys it becomes a form of vitamin D. Like an astute oil company, the body tightly regulates the supply of refined products in the body's metabolic economy. For example, when the body has enough testosterone, the testes cut back on their production through a feedback loop. But what would happen if this feedback were disrupted? The cholesterol products would accumulate excessively. A person would develop a hormone glut.

Something like this happened to the Raskins' baby. A particularly complex refinery called the adrenal gland covers the kidneys like a beret. From cholesterol, the adrenal gland makes—among other hormones—the key substance cortisol. As with testosterone, cortisol levels are regulated by a feedback loop. That's where the problem was: our patient couldn't make cortisol. Sensing a deficit of cortisol, the body kept forcing the adrenal to make hormones. But no cortisol ever came. The adrenal gland just kept making the only cholesterol-based hormone it *could* make: an analogue of testosterone. Though female, the baby experienced a glut of male hormone that enlarged her clitoris so that it looked like a small penis. This condition is called congenital adrenal hyperplasia, or CAH. The lab had called to tell us that the baby had abnormal levels of cortisol-type hormones, making the diagnosis.

An endocrine specialist went to explain our findings to the Raskins. Evan Stringer and I spoke again at the baby's bedside and wrote orders to begin cortisol hormones by mouth. This would satisfy the baby's need and reduce the signal for continued adrenal hormone production. The male hormones would go back to normal levels, for a female.

I reached for a pink card and began to fill it out with the words "Raskin, Baby Girl." The endocrinologist recommended surgical remodeling of the genitals to a more female form. Her other blood test, when it returned, confirmed that she had two X-chromosomes. In some way, this released some tension: the baby finally had a sexual identity.

But did she?

In 1975, Anke Ehrhardt compared seventeen patients like Baby Girl Raskin to their healthy sisters to study their gender identity. All the patients had had surgery to appear female and took replacement hormones by mouth, just as we had recommended for our patient. The results of Ehrhardt's follow-up were fascinating. The younger CAH patients preferred boys as playmates half the time, compared to less than 5 percent of the time for their healthy sisters. While almost all the normal siblings played with dolls, less than one in ten of the CAH patients did. The differences persisted well into adolescence; 60 percent of the CAH patients were "tomboyish" and also had no interest in jewelry and makeup, compared to less than 10 percent of their siblings. A 1984 study found that only 40 percent of adult women with CAH said they were "exclusively heterosexual," and that 35 percent were "bisexual or homosexual."

This information demonstrates the complexity of gender assignment. Though these girls and women with CAH had two X-chromosomes, ovaries, externally female genitals, and adequate levels of female hormones, they continued to have characteristics societally viewed as male, perhaps due to their prenatal exposure to male hormones. How, then, should maleness and femaleness be defined? Psychologists today view gender as a collection of five independent qualities: genetic makeup, external appearance, brain organization, sexual orientation, and personal gender identity. Thus, a typical woman is female in all areas. A person with CAH, however, may have female genes, external appearance, and gender identity, but a male brain organization and sexual orientation. A person with "gender dysphoria," that is, someone who might seek a sex-change operation, may be a particular sex in all matters except gender identity. A gay man, for example, might be male in all aspects except sexual orientation.

In a sense, children like Baby Girl Raskin challenge our tendency to simplify complex psychological and medical phenomena. Her future, though likely one that will be metabolically healthy, will not be easy. To function in society, she will likely have to pigeonhole herself into a gender role that may confine her true nature. How might her playmates treat a girl who doesn't like dolls, or her peer group a tomboyish teenage girl with little interest in clothing or makeup? How will her parents react if she is a lesbian? Will she, by some measure, remain true to herself, and even if she does, how will the world respond to her?

I think it's unlikely that the determinants of gender identity will ever be fully catalogued, at least enough to adequately predict a baby's future orientation based on blood tests or brain scans or something comparable. These factors mirror those involved in predicting love, which depends so nebulously on unique situations, metaphors, culture, society, and preferences inherited in some fashion—be it by genes or upbringing—from one's parents and community.

Before my father died, he once called me into his room and pointed to a locked filing cabinet. In it, he housed his financial papers, various contracts, and other documents. Acutely aware of his poor health status, he had previously discussed financial arrangements with me in case of medical catastrophe, so I knew where to find his will and how to contact his lawyer. It had been an unpleasant but necessary conversation.

Today, he wanted to talk about love, not abstractly, but about his love for my mother. We had rarely seen eye-to-eye about love. By arrangement, his own father was married while a teenager to a barely pubescent girl in a remote Indian village. Romantic love, my grandfather said once, was an unmentionable topic that threatened the fabric of orderly Indian society. The marriages of each of his six sons were arranged, and my father's was no exception. While in his twenties, my father was introduced to my mother. After a single meeting, in which the two drank pepper-laced pomegranate juice at Bombay's Chowpatty Beach, he decided to marry her. Having grown up in suburban America, I found this type of courtship incomprehensible. Once in a while I poked fun at my father's approach to love, for what did he know of romance?

That day he talked about how he wanted my mother cared for, if he died. He told me how they had met and grown together. And he finally pointed to a green file that hung in the back of his cabinet. "You might," he said, "want to read this someday after I die. But not now." He didn't say what was in the file. He closed the drawer and locked it with a small gold key.

Some weeks after my father's death, I went to the cabinet and unlocked it with the key, which he had left for me. I slid open the drawer and retrieved the green file. I took it to a reading desk and opened it.

The folder was full of letters arranged in chronological order, written in my father's crisp print on yellowed sheets of paper. The pages were addressed to my mother, beginning shortly after he met her. Though he barely knew her, he had fallen for her immediately. The pages were love letters. "I have always been something of a vagabond," he wrote in his first letter, "and I would like to share the world with you." In simple but exquisite prose, he wrote letter after letter, constructing and decorating a love for a woman he had barely met, and while reading I realized that, despite his upbringing, something in him—who knew what—had fashioned him into a closet romantic. He was true to himself. I wondered why he shared the letters with me, and supposed he wanted someone to know that he had loved with intensity, mentioning to me what was unmentionable to one's children during his own youth.

Guts

ON REMEDYING VARIOUS KINDS OF EMPTINESS,
AND A CONCLUDING CONFESSION

The one-month-old boy's skin was surprisingly elastic, like dough. I bent over the table in the emergency room and gently pinched his thigh. Like a little tent, the skin remained propped up after I removed my fingers; this was worrisome.

The mystery of how flour mixed with water becomes dough was recently solved by a chemist from Kansas, and has some relevance for the one-month-old. When hydrated, two proteins in flour called gliadin and glutenin swell like sponges, and cling to form a material called gluten. As it ferments flour, yeast releases carbon dioxide, which partially inflates the porous gluten like a half-full hot-air balloon. Thus dough rises, but not so much so that it becomes tense. Like the baby's skin, it can be molded.

Typically, baby skin cells are so full that they're as firm as basket-balls; it's only when they become depleted that they seem elastic. The baby had the opposite condition as rising dough: instead of being filled, his skin cells were being emptied. The healthy human body contains roughly 70 percent water, but this baby's percentage was far lower. His skin was elastic because he was profoundly dehydrated.

Such dehydration brings the body to a grinding halt. The loss of water causes the blood volume to contract. Though the heart struggles to respond by pumping harder and faster, it eventually can't keep up. That makes the blood pressure fall, and the body becomes starved for oxygen. Without oxygen the heating system fails, and one's temperature drops degree by degree. An affected baby begins dying. Worldwide, three million children are lost in this fashion every year, but this boy wasn't going to be one of them.

We placed the child on a warmer and hooked him up to a monitor. His heart was going like a hummingbird's wings, so fast that I could barely tell when one beat ended and the next began. He was breathing, but seemed very tired. The main priority was getting some fluid into him. To insert an IV, two experienced nurses tied tourniquets on the boy's arms and tried to catch any veins that might appear. None did, since the boy was so dehydrated that his veins just didn't fill.

There was only one alternative: an intraosseous line, or IO. I called for one, and a nurse placed it in my hand. The thickness of a sewing needle, an IO infuses liquid directly into a person's bone. Within the center or marrow of many bones, such as the thigh and calf bones, there are large blood vessels. These can be reached once an IO needle is pushed through the bone. This isn't a delicate procedure. Using a brown antiseptic soap, I sterilized the skin over the infant's calf, and after mustering strength, twisted the IO like a corkscrew into the baby's leg. The nurses connected a bag of saline fluid to the IO and squeezed it to force fluid into the baby's circulation. We waited.

In the meantime, the paramedics reported that the child's name was Edwin Skeets, and he'd had diarrhea for several days. Edwin's mother added that his diapers overflowed with brownish water almost ten times that day. She tried to breast-feed him, but her milk just couldn't keep up. Edwin looked as if he was deflating, she said.

Generally, the average infant passes a half-teaspoon's worth of stool daily for every pound of weight. That averages to a tablespoon per day for a newborn. By three years of age, a child achieves adult stool volume, which is about three ounces a day. Stool production of more than twice the normal amount is called diarrhea. Because Edwin passed over twenty times the usual amount of stool, which is made mostly of water, he rapidly became dehydrated.

Following food through the gut helps to understand Edwin's problem. Swallowed nutrients enter the stomach, a gourd-shaped chamber a few inches below the left nipple. There—like a car entering an automatic washing station—the food is bathed in water, agitated, and scrubbed by the rhythmic churning of the stomach. Substances made in the saliva and stomach process the food, breaking the starches into sugar and cracking proteins into amino acids. From the stomach, the contents are squirted in small portions into the duodenum, the portal to the small intestine.

There, as in the second phase of a car wash, detergents (which break up fat) and digestive enzymes are added by the liver and pancreas. Including the amount taken by mouth and also secreted so far, about two and a half gallons of fluid enter the average child's duodenum daily. At this point, the breaking up of food into smaller components is largely finished. Completing the final drying phase of the wash cycle, the food travels through the twelve feet of the small intestine. During this trip, nutrients and 90 percent of the water are absorbed into the bloodstream.

That's where Edwin had problems. Absorption depends on surface area. For example, a geographic area with numerous hills and valleys requires much more rain to saturate the ground than a flat region of the same acreage does. The former terrain has a lot more area to cover. The small intestine takes advantage of this principle. Resembling a shag carpet, it's lined with tens of millions of microscopic, fingerlike projections called villi that expand the surface area of the small intestine enormously, from less than two square feet to the area of a tennis court. Villi absorb nutrients and water very efficiently.

Something disabled Edwin's villi so they couldn't absorb his food and water. Instead of permitting only 10 percent of the stomach contents to pass to the end of the small intestine, Edwin let almost all of it through. From there, the deluge went into the large intestine, which doesn't absorb as well as the small intestine. The large intestine passed the material on through like an overwhelmed dam, causing diarrhea.

To become severely dehydrated, an infant needs to lose about 15 percent of his weight. For Edwin, that was about a half-quart of water that we'd have to replace quickly. In perspective, it's like an average adult losing two to three gallons of fluid. As we pumped saline into Edwin's bone, I wondered what had attacked the boy's villi.

Most likely, Edwin had some kind of infection. One possibility was *Shigella*, the second most common cause of bacterial diarrhea in American children. The great physician William Osler called it "one of the great four epidemic diseases of the world." After taking up residence in the small intestine, *Shigella* makes a poison that kills villi and makes them leak water. It is so potent that a *single gram* of feces from an infected person has enough bacteria to poison every person in the state of Pennsylvania, and a complete bowel movement has enough organisms to infect every last American citizen.

Another possibility was *Salmonella*, which is more common than *Shigella* but has a similar effect on the small intestine. After people recover from *Salmonella* infection, they can be contagious carriers for years, without any symptoms. This lesson was learned in the early twentieth century, when the well-appearing Irish immigrant Mary Mallon refused to abandon her cooking jobs, despite infecting over fifty people with traces of her stool and earning herself the appellation Typhoid Mary (the eponymous fever is caused by a type of *Salmonella*). After a dramatic flight into a forest, she was captured by police and imprisoned for life in a hospital outside New York.

Salmonella's sordid saga continued in 1984, when in Wasco County, Oregon, it was used in history's first bioterrorist attack against Americans. Members of the Bhagwan Shree Rajneesh cult purchased the organism from the Maryland-based American Type Culture Collection (the same source from which Iraqi agents may have obtained anthrax for weaponization), cultivated it in a make-shift lab, and used it to contaminate salad bars at restaurants on the eve of a local election. Almost 750 people developed diarrhea. Only after a year of study did federal authorities realize what had occurred.

Salmonella can be acquired in less dramatic ways; for example, the U.S. Department of Agriculture reports that 30 percent of ground turkey and 15 percent of ground chicken in meat-processing plants contain the organism. Thus, pediatricians always recommend that meats given to children be thoroughly cooked. Certain animals, such as reptiles, also carry the microbe. In 1996, sixty-five children developed *Salmonella* infection after petting a Komodo dragon at a zoo, leading to calls to limit hands-on exhibits involving reptiles.

There are also other diarrhea-causing bacteria like *E. coli*, which caused a notorious outbreak from undercooked hamburgers made by the Jack-in-the-Box fast-food chain. However, none of these seemed responsible for Edwin's dehydration. He lacked the telltale bloody stools. He didn't have a fever, and his blood counts didn't suggest bacterial infection. There were other, more likely, possibilities.

So far, we'd pumped nine ounces—maybe three Dixie cups' worth—of saline into Edwin, and he was looking better. In addition to having elastic skin, dehydrated children have dry mouths, lack tears when they cry, urinate minimally, and seem very tired. After getting the saline, Edwin did urinate and also appeared more awake.

"What have you been feeding your baby?" I asked Edwin's mother. Only breast milk, she replied. About 2 percent of children have allergies to cow's milk, present in formula or in the breast milk of mothers who drink a lot of cow's milk. The immune system in a baby's gut attacks ingested cow's milk, and villi at the site of the attack sustain collateral damage. Diarrhea results, which usually resolves two days after milk is eliminated from the diet because healthy villi grow back. The long-term prognosis of milk allergy is favorable, since three-quarters of affected children are no longer allergic by six years of age. However, Edwin's mother said she didn't drink much cow's milk, making the diagnosis unlikely.

Could Edwin be lactose intolerant? Like cow's milk, breast milk contains lots of lactose, a type of sugar. Adults who get bloating, diarrhea, or cramping after ingesting milk products can't digest the sugar. It's a fascinating problem. No human can absorb lactose unless it's broken down into smaller pieces. Therefore, in every baby's small intestine, the tips of the villi have little scissors called lactases, which perform this task and allow babies to absorb lactose pieces. For unknown reasons, these scissors on the villi disappear in three-quarters of adults. In these individuals, lactose passes whole into the large intestine, which normally teems with bacteria. The cornucopia of sugar is a festive treat for these bacteria, which release loads of hydrogen gas as they feast. This is exceedingly uncomfortable for the party's host, who feels like a large balloon is suddenly inflated within the bowels. (There are even reports of operating-room explosions during gastrointestinal surgery in lactose intolerant people exposed to cauterizing instruments, which ignited the hydrogen.) As a final insult, lactose draws excess water into the large intestine, and causes diarrhea. However, lactose intolerance bad enough to cause Edwin's degree of dehydration is extraordinarily rare in newborns.

Almost certainly, Edwin's intestines were infected with rotavirus, the most common cause of diarrhea in children today and the second most prevalent illness after the common cold. Resembling a tire with spokes radiating from a hub (*rota* is Latin for wheel), the virus destroys the villi of the small intestine. Most American children get infected at some time before their second birthday, and the diarrhea can last a week. This hunch was later confirmed by a test of Edwin's stool, which was positive for rotavirus parts.

Today, most parents in the United States see diarrhea as an annoyance; the average family absorbs about $300 in extra day-care costs and lost wages every time a child gets the condition. But as Edwin's case suggests, diarrhea can also have worse consequences. Every year, 200,000 American infants are hospitalized for diarrhea and 500 die of dehydration. Worldwide, *millions* of children die of diarrhea each year, a number that would be even higher were it not for a discovery stemming from an ancient plague called cholera.

Cholera originated in areas around India's Ganges River, which by legend flows from the hair of Shiva, the Hindu deity of destruction. Since the early 1800s, seven global pandemics of cholera have occurred, most recently in 1991 when 400,000 cases appeared in Latin America. The plague even entered America. From illegally shipped crab's meat, eight people in New Jersey also caught the ailment, not far from where I grew up.

In infected people, the organism disperses through the small intestine and makes a toxin that reverses the gut's absorption of water. Instead of removing water from the small intestine, the poisoned villi pump water into the small intestine. The resulting diarrhea is extraordinary. In some countries, sufferers lay on wooden beds with a hole cut around the buttocks, and experience watery bowel movements lasting days. Cholera, though, is not particularly hard to fight off, and a person's immune system dispatches the invaders in a few days. The key is staying hydrated until then, and there are several ways to do this.

Like Edwin, a dehydrated child could get fluids pumped directly into the veins. A simple salt mixture usually suffices, but many places can't afford these sterile solutions. In Malaysia, an interesting discovery was made: coconut milk, which is also sterile, can be injected directly into the veins. Thus in some poor areas, coconuts take the place of intravenous bags. But many areas also lack coconuts.

In these locations, one might think, children could just drink lots of water. But this doesn't help, since children with cholera also lose up to twenty teaspoons of salt daily in the stool. In fact, these children get very thirsty and can drink gallons of plain water. This instinct is dangerous, since excessive water consumption dilutes the remaining salt in the bloodstream, causing seizures, brain swelling, and problems with heart rhythms.

In the 1950s, doctors figured that a beverage with the same salt concentrations as diarrhea might fix a child's dual deficit of water and salt. Since it would be cheaper to produce and give (no needles or sterile components were required), the drink might work in poor areas. But it didn't: although a child took up the water readily from the small intestine, sodium molecules in the salt remained behind like wallflowers. A remarkable—and exceedingly simple—insight followed. In 1964, R. Phillips found that glucose (a kind of sugar) could pair up with salt, and the couple together could be absorbed very efficiently from the small intestine. Glucose was the missing partner that salt needed. In the mid-1970s, the World Health Organization agreed that oral rehydration solution, or ORS, should contain equal parts glucose and sodium. (A homemade recipe for ORS is to add one teaspoon of salt, three tablespoons of sugar, and one cup of orange juice to three cups of water.) Children drinking ORS replenished both their water and salt deficits, and survived through the days of severe diarrhea. In a triumph for public health, fatality rates from cholera epidemics fell dramatically from almost 25 percent to less than 1 percent where packets of powdered ORS were distributed.

Not far from where Edwin became ill, the Asian Indian–born researcher Mathuram Santosham wondered if ORS could be used for diarrheal illnesses other than cholera. A remarkable man, Santosham has performed many health studies in Navajo and Apache country and overcome a long-standing distrust of medical research. At his first meeting with tribal officials, he was asked whether he could identify with Native Americans. He quipped, "Why, yes. If Columbus had known his geography, *I'd* be living on a reservation and you'd want to study *me*." In a 1985 study in Whiteriver, Arizona, Santosham convincingly showed that 98 percent of diarrhea cases (including those from rotavirus) in children could be managed with ORS instead of expensive intravenous fluids.

After being stabilized in the emergency room, Edwin was admitted to the pediatric ward. I removed his intraosseous line, since its continued presence could cause an infection in the bone. I prescribed an ORS solution called Rehydralyte and specified the target amounts Edwin should drink. His mother took a feeding syringe and placed one teaspoonful in Edwin's mouth every few minutes. At that rate, her son would be fully replenished in a day.

Interestingly, many people still believe that a clear liquid diet is best during diarrhea. This is erroneous. For example, chicken broth has twice as much salt and less than one-hundredth the amount of glucose as ORS. Apple juice contains seven times the amount of sugar, and less than one-hundredth the amount of salt as ORS. Interestingly, the "scientifically formulated" sports drink Gatorade has made serious accommodations in the name of palatability, since the average serving has over twice the amount of sugar and one-quarter the amount of salt as ORS. For infants with serious dehydration, no beverages other than specifically designed ORS solutions like Rehydralyte, Pedialyte, or Infalyte are appropriate. Finally, a regular diet should be resumed within twenty-four hours.

After about two days, Edwin was back to normal. His tenting, wizened skin became supple, and he'd regained his chubby looks. I completed his discharge paperwork and said good-bye. A few hours later, I spied his mother and him at the local gas station. Edwin's mother waved and returned to filling her four-by-four's tank for the long trip back to their home on the reservation.

Edwin had a problem transporting nutrients from the small intestine into the blood. Eight-year-old Taylor Briscoe, however, had a slightly different crisis. After eating and absorbing her meal, Taylor couldn't get the nutrients from her blood to go into her body's cells. That's why her breath smelled so fruity.

Taylor's parents brought their daughter to the emergency room at Children's Hospital because she had been losing weight for a few weeks, although she always seemed to be eating. A gray-eyed, fresh-faced girl, Taylor wore denim overalls that seemed too big. "They used to fit well," her mother said, frowning.

Rapid weight loss in a child is very worrisome, and can be explained by one of two conditions. First, a child—or something inside her body—could be using up too much energy. A rapidly growing tumor or some intestinal parasite could be stealing Taylor's glucose. A child could be fighting an exhausting battle with a hidden infection, like tuberculosis or even HIV. Or the heart could be failing from some infection or genetic problem. Getting through a routine day for these individuals is as tiring as running a marathon, and weight loss invariably results.

The other possibility was that Taylor wasn't getting enough nutrition. For example, she could have developed an allergy to gluten, the substance responsible for bread's rising. Called "celiac disease," this illness causes intestinal swelling that interferes with nutrient absorption. She could have cystic fibrosis (the same disease that Bobby Aire and Peter West had in the chapter about lungs), which prohibits the release of digestive substances in the intestines. Perhaps, even, she was secretly dieting.

"Taylor's always thirsty and always going to the bathroom. A few days ago, she wet her pants in the car," said the girl's mother, and Taylor looked at the floor in embarrassment. This was an important clue. With Taylor's urine and a group of ants, a physician could have determined her diagnosis.

This isn't as unusual as it sounds. After eating, a child absorbs sugar from the small intestine. As if coming through international customs, all blood from the small intestine passes through a checkpoint, the liver. Located slightly below the right nipple, the liver is the body's largest internal organ. There, the nutrient-rich blood percolates through cells called hepatocytes, which set how much glucose may pass on to the body.

Just as the lungs manage oxygen in the blood, the liver regulates glucose in the blood. This is a critical task. Like oxygen, glucose is so vital that its depletion—even for a few minutes—can cause irreversible brain damage or other organ failure. Like oxygen, glucose isn't present in large amounts. The average person's blood has only a few tablespoons at a given time, not enough to power the body for very long. Just as the lungs must breathe oxygen into the body continuously, the liver breathes sugar into the bloodstream.

The organ that tells the liver when to "inhale" and "exhale" sugar (so to speak) is the pancreas, found next to the stomach. Like an investment bank, the liver deposits glucose absorbed from the intestines into a secure fund called glycogen. Under very high magnification, stores of glycogen appear like coin-shaped granules in liver cells.

The pancreas calls on the liver to make withdrawals from this account. When a child like Taylor hasn't eaten in a while, the body's glucose gets used up, and the pancreas asks the liver to put sugar into the blood. For example, the body's glucose currency is used overnight during sleep, so the liver releases enough to ensure that the body continues to function. It "exhales" glucose.

Similarly, when there is abundant glucose in the blood, the pancreas tells the liver and the body to absorb glucose, or "inhale." But what happens when the pancreas doesn't do this job? The bloodstream overflows with sugar, which spills into the urine, which normally contains no sugar. The sugar drags along a lot of water, so the body passes large amounts of sugary urine.

Taylor almost certainly had this illness. Thousands of years ago, ancient Hindu physicians described a strange, deadly condition of wasting and intense thirst, in which the sufferer's urine attracted ants and flies. In 250 B.C., Apollonius of Memphis coined the modern name for the disease, which literally means "to go through," describing what Greek physicians called the "melting down of the flesh and limbs into urine."

Taylor climbed up on the exam table, and I looked at her hands to place her at ease. They were normal. "What grade are you in?" I asked, and when she answered, I noticed that her breath had a vague, citrus-and-apple odor. "Did you just eat some candy or an orange?" I asked. "No," said Taylor. The rest of her exam was normal. Because some blood tests needed to be sent, I had Taylor lie on her back and tied a tourniquet around her arm. Several plump blood vessels appeared. "Will this hurt?" she asked, fearfully.

Physicians inexperienced with children answer this question wrong. "Yes," they say truthfully, "but it'll hurt only for a few seconds." Many children—especially toddlers and early school age kids—can't comprehend time scales; they only process the words "yes" and "hurt." Screaming usually ensues. The well-meaning doctors compound their initial error by counting down to the moment of pain. "Look how small this needle is," they say, and display the syringe. Then they recite, "We're ready to go on three. Ready? One . . . two . . . three!" This strategy focuses all of the child's attention on the dreaded moment, amplifying their fear by orders of magnitude. For an already unglued patient, a simple procedure becomes intensely traumatic.

I resort to telling some white lies. "I don't know if it hurts," I said to Taylor. "Some people think it feels warm, and some people think it feels really icy." I hid the syringe from view with my hands. A nurse distracted the child with conversation and a picture book. I chatted aimlessly, and between words quickly inserted the needle. (I rarely use a countdown, but when I do, I tell the child I'll count down from ten to one and somewhat dishonestly stick in the needle at seven.)

Taylor barely flinched, and I withdrew a tablespoon of blood. Though bandages are generally unnecessary, I put one on Taylor anyway. The blood and a sample of Taylor's urine were sent to the lab, and I waited at the nursing station for the results. They came back in a few minutes, and confirmed the diagnosis.

It's strange knowing something nobody else does, especially when the knowledge could change someone's life forever. Several years ago, for example, a genetic test to determine whether a person would get Huntington's chorea (the condition affecting folk musician Woody Guthrie) was invented. The disease is uniformly fatal after a long deterioration of one's body, and there is no treatment. Someone born to an affected person, like Woody Guthrie's son Arlo, has a 50 percent chance of getting Huntington's chorea, which develops in early adulthood. The uncertainty is haunting, and some people want to know their fate. "The devil you know is far better than the one you don't know," said one person who requested testing for the gene. Arlo Guthrie, on the other hand, preferred never to get checked. (Now over fifty years old, he seems not to have the illness.)

Ergun Uc, an Arkansas specialist on Huntington's chorea, finds that half of people who do get tested decide—after the mandatory one-month waiting period before the results can be accessed—that they really *don't* want to know their fate. Only the few technicians running the tests know their results, and never divulge them. I think this secret knowledge must be a great burden. One lab worker said he often fantasized about calling people with negative tests to disclose the good news. I'd probably have the same desire.

In Taylor's case, the life-changing lab results weren't to remain secret. The final moments of the family's ignorance passed while I walked back to their exam room. I opened the door, entered, and began a long discussion about Taylor's problem, which was diabetes.

Taylor's pancreas wasn't working right. Though rightly telling the liver when to "exhale" glucose via the hormone glucagon, the pancreas wasn't getting the liver to "inhale" glucose because it couldn't make the hormone insulin. The pancreas had been smoldering for a year, since almost 98 percent of the insulin-producing cells must die before diabetes occurs. Nobody knows why this happens; the body's immune system somehow gets confused and attacks these innocent cells. These so-called autoimmune conditions are common; for example, the main reason physicians prescribe penicillin for strep throat is to prevent autoimmune damage to a heart valve (rheumatic fever), not to improve the sore throat.

Unfortunately, as with strep throat and rheumatic fever, there is no known preceding infection that heralds diabetes. No preventable risk factors have been identified, although in the 1970s, a rat poison called Vacor was pulled from the market after several children accidentally ingested it and developed diabetes. Today, diabetic children typically present like Taylor, with weight loss, excessive thirst and urination, and fruity breath. By then, the pancreas is already damaged beyond repair. Lab tests show very high levels of glucose in body fluids and a remarkable acidity in the blood that causes fruity breath.

Taylor's body had a glucose crisis akin to a financial panic. After a normal child eats, insulin promotes the saving of glucose into glycogen accounts in the liver. However, due to an absence of insulin, Taylor couldn't invest her glucose for later use; it all stayed in her blood. Problematically, her pancreas continued making glucagon, which caused her liver to liquidate her glycogen stores. A rapid sell-off of her assets occurred. The excess of glucose in Taylor's blood overwhelmed her kidneys, which lost the valuable assets in the urine. Her body experienced a depression; there was no energy left for everyday activities, let alone growth. Thus, Taylor lost weight.

Glucagon also forced Taylor to tap her rainy-day fund: fat. Her liver processed fat into acidic molecules called ketones, an energy source usable by the brain and certain other organs. Some ketones vaporize within the lungs, giving the breath its characteristic fruity odor. While ketones are a good alternative fuel, high levels increase blood acidity excessively, and place the entire body in jeopardy. Taylor's blood was in fact acidic, and her ketone levels were so high that she spilled them in her urine and breath. Untreated, Taylor would eventually suffer the "melting down" into urine described by ancient Greeks. Therefore, I admitted her to the hospital and called a diabetes specialist for advice. Together, we plotted to turn around her metabolic depression.

A century ago, the average child diagnosed with diabetes could expect to live only one year. Around that time, researchers discovered that dogs without a pancreas developed diabetes. By 1920, a method for purifying insulin from canine pancreatic tissue was developed. The first patient to receive insulin, a rail-thin fourteen-year-old named Leonard Thompson, got an injection of three teaspoons of "thick brown muck"—the dog extract—into his buttocks. A miraculous recovery followed, and with regular injections Thompson gained weight and survived for many years. The life expectancy for diabetics treated with insulin soon soared. Today, commercially available insulin is produced by genetically engineered bacteria, not dogs, but is still given by injection.

In the hospital, Taylor began a crash course on diabetes care. Her life would never be the same. Each day, a steady stream of dieticians, endocrinologists, social workers, and nurses tutored Taylor on her new responsibilities. From now on, she'd have to do what her pancreas formerly did, which is control her blood sugar.

The body performs the most complex regulatory feats automatically, and most of us take if for granted. The act of walking, for example, seems simple enough. Yet when we stand, the brain makes the heart pump faster, and veins in the legs constrict to push extra blood into the circulation. Balance sensors in the ear ensure the brain tightens and loosens various muscles to prevent falling. The pancreas may release glucagon, so that adequate energy stores are mobilized. One breathes slightly harder. The list goes on and on. It's a good thing this activity occurs unconsciously; if it didn't, we'd think of nothing else. Even assuming the responsibilities of a single organ—such as the pancreas—can be overwhelming.

Taylor had little room for error. If her glucose levels become too high, she'd over time damage her eyes, kidneys, and heart, and develop blood acidity that could be fatal. If levels were too low, she'd experience hypoglycemia, characterized by fatigue, sweating, and, possibly, organ damage. The body's control of glucose can be compared to the Federal Reserve Bank's control of interest rates, where small changes in the availability of a resource (whether money or glucose) are used to make major changes (whether in a national economy or in the body), and a small error can cause big problems. To cope with her diabetes, Taylor had to learn some metabolic economics.

The first lesson was the hardest. The morning after admission, a nurse and I went to Taylor's room and sat down with the family. We'd already talked about what Taylor needed to do. She took a little needle from her blood sugar testing kit and attached it to a spring-loaded guillotine-like device the size of a matchbox. "You can do it," said Taylor's mother, squeezing her daughter's hand.

Taylor put the guillotine over her right index finger and squeezed her eyes shut. Little wrinkles appeared on her forehead and, with a little cry, she clicked the loaded device with her left hand. I heard a little snap as the needle pricked Taylor's finger. A small drop of bright red blood appeared. "You did it!" exclaimed Taylor's father.

Just as we had explained, Taylor took the blood and put it on the glucometer, a wallet-sized machine that started counting down from thirty on a liquid crystal screen. After a half-minute, the glucometer beeped and displayed a number, 175, which was the blood glucose level. Overnight, the nurses had checked Taylor's glucose; this was the first time the child performed it herself. We congratulated her.

Now came the more difficult part. As we had shown her, Taylor took an alcohol wipe and cleaned the top of a vial of insulin. Then she took a syringe, removed its protective cap, plunged the needle into the vial, and extracted a precise amount of the drug. Her concentration was impressive; I didn't even see her blink. "Are you ready to do this?" asked Taylor's nurse. The girl nodded and clenched her teeth. She cleaned a little patch of skin on her belly with alcohol, pinched it, and inserted the needle into the fold. After flinching slightly, she pressed the syringe to inject the insulin, and pulled out the needle. The nurse and I smiled broadly. "You were great!" I said. Though she didn't smile, she did nod.

Overnight, the nurses had given all the shots, but now Taylor would have to do her own shots. For the rest of her life, Taylor would have to check her blood sugar and give herself the medication, sometimes five times a day.

The next lessons involved exchange rates, covering the carbohydrate contents of various foods and appropriate doses of insulin. Taylor's daily diet was painfully specific: She'd be allowed sixteen calories per pound she weighed, and take a fifth of this at breakfast, a fifth at lunch, slightly more at dinner, and the rest at three specific snacks. When these limits were exceeded, more insulin was needed.

A dietician helped Taylor and her parents understand how to count calories in foods, and calculate "carbohydrate equivalents." For every fifteen extra grams of carbohydrates eaten, Taylor had to inject one extra unit of insulin. The family caught on well. On the second day, I watched the dietician drill them using flashcards of foods, and Taylor and her parents crisply identified the carbohydrate equivalents.

Taylor was ready to go home after two days. A stack of pamphlets about diabetes sat at her bedside. Several follow-up appointments were made to reinforce proper care, and Taylor signed up for a summer "diabetes camp" for children, where recreational activities were mingled with educational ones. (These camps are present nationwide; in fact, the campground where I volunteered as a counselor for children with cancer was owned by the American Diabetes Association and usually hosted children with diabetes.)

Before her discharge, I kept Taylor company while her parents ran some errands. She seemed a little wistful. "They said I can't have cake at birthday parties," she reported, "and I like cake." In the hospital, some of her friends had brought candy, not knowing that she couldn't eat it. "I had to give it all to my sister," she said, looking at her hands.

Like many children with chronic or life-threatening illnesses, Taylor acutely felt the loss of normalcy. In 1969, psychiatrist Elisabeth Kübler-Ross published *On Death and Dying*, ending a profound silence from physicians about the process of grieving. Kübler-Ross identified five stages—denial, anger, bargaining, depression, and acceptance—that grieving adults go through sequentially. Children, however, rarely follow this orderly pattern. Like Taylor, some seem immediately to accept a diagnosis, and only later experience anger or sadness. Some young children view illness or death as temporary conditions (occasionally confused by adult terminology like "Your mother had to go to sleep") and grieve for briefer or more intermittent periods than adults. Because they have difficulty articulating their feelings, children may act out through aggressive actions, school phobia, or loss of toileting skills.

In general, I think that just as a child's body regulates glucose through unconscious mechanisms, a child's psyche regulates his or her grief in a complex but ultimately sensible manner. In the absence of something obviously pathological, which is uncommon, I let children determine the cadence and intensity of their grief. Thus, I didn't approach Taylor and pressure her to talk about her feelings. I didn't try to elicit denial or anger, in the hope that their expression would be healthy. I just made myself available and listened.

Taylor talked about things she would miss eating, and then changed the subject. "The nurse said I'd gain weight back soon, and my mom said she'd take me shopping to get some new clothes," she said, and smiled.

The deficiencies of Taylor Briscoe and the dehydrated child Edwin Skeets expose an interesting irony. What each child lacked was already within the body, tantalizingly close but inaccessible. The sugar in Taylor's blood was there for the taking; her body just had to request it with insulin. Similarly, Edwin could absorb all the salt he needed from his gut; he just needed some sugar in the oral hydration solution.

Unlike them, sixteen-year-old Meg Parsons had no problems absorbing, storing, or distributing what she ate. In fact, food was there for the taking and her gut was entirely healthy, which is why her nutritional deficiency was the most ironic problem of all.

Like Taylor, Meg was brought to the emergency room for treatment of her rapid weight loss. A muscular, scrub-clad orderly stood guard at the door to her room. I entered and noted that Meg's breath smelled fine. The girl's stringy hair framed a thin face. When Meg's half-lidded eyes sometimes opened wide as we talked, they had a haunted, burning look.

This wasn't the first time, or even the second or third, that Meg had been in this situation. Her exhausted parents leaned against the wall in her room, looking at the floor. While talking, I flipped through the chart, noting that Meg weighed eighty pounds, down fifteen from her last admission several months ago. That time, she once asked to go to the bathroom, and disappeared. Security barely caught her near the hospital's main entrance, which is why an orderly guarded her door now.

Today the heart rate was forty beats per minute, about half of mine. Her body temperature was also two degrees lower than normal. These numbers indicated a state of starvation, like that present in a prisoner of war or hibernating animal. Unlike Taylor's body, which reacted to nutrient deprivation with intense hunger pangs and a rapid heart rate, Meg's body was so used to the chronic deficit that it simply slowed itself down and adapted. Meg wasn't even hungry.

This is the body's normal response to prolonged starvation. In 1990, for example, a researcher placed a group of obese patients on a highly restricted diet, which permitted only 200 calories—the amount roughly in a 12-ounce can of soda—daily. After three weeks, the subjects didn't salivate after being shown slides of food and had almost no hunger. In another study on patients with Meg's specific problem, the smell and sight of a cinnamon roll caused subjects to release hormones associated with hunger; however, the patients had no desire to eat the roll. It appears that certain starved people can prohibit stimuli, such as the presence of food or even specific hormones, from triggering hunger.

As usual, I began an exam by looking at Meg's hands, which were cool and slightly dry. There were some calluses on her knuckles, and some small healing cuts. Sadly, this was to be expected, especially because her cheeks had a swollen, chipmunk look. Listening to the heart, I could barely get my stethoscope to lie flat, since Meg was so thin that her ribs protruded like train tracks. Under her baggy sleeves, I noted that her arms grew fine hair called lanugo, like that present on some newborn babys' arms and backs.

Meg's problem was "anorexia nervosa," and she had been sick for three years. The fundamental problem in anorexia is that a person has both a delusion that she is overweight and an obsession to be thinner, beliefs that are unchanged by any degree of weight loss.

Among girls, the desire to be thin isn't unusual; surveys show that more than half of all adolescent girls are trying to lose weight. Many of them have distorted body images; a Canadian study found that 80 percent of girls thinking they were too fat actually had normal body weights. From a young age, children are surrounded by images of thinness; for example, if Mattel's Barbie doll were a standard female height, her waist would be 18 inches. Today, the average female magazine model is a size 2. To achieve this idealized thinness, almost one in ten adolescent girls takes diet pills, and one in five college-age women has vomited intentionally at least once to lose weight.

Anorexic girls like Meg, however, go to extraordinary lengths to become thin. On her chart, previous residents documented that Meg had a long history of "purging" after meals. She'd go to the bathroom and stick her finger down her throat to vomit. Like many anorexics, she did this frequently enough that her teeth decayed slightly from stomach acid, and her fingers developed scrapes and calluses from rubbing against her teeth. Because she lost so much saliva and stomach acid, the glands producing saliva near her cheeks expanded, to keep up with demand. (This explained her "chipmunk" face.) She secretly took large doses of laxatives to flush out her gut, obviating its normal absorption. Her mother noticed that Meg's sneakers wore out quickly, and later discovered Meg was running stairs in her house for hours every night after everyone was asleep.

Like alcoholics, anorexics have a disease characterized by periods of stability followed by periods of relapse. Meg had fallen off the wagon some weeks ago and resumed her weight-losing behaviors. I felt a desire to say, "Look at yourself. Why don't you just eat?" but refrained. The care of such patients is intensely frustrating to me; rational maneuvers like showing a low body-mass index on a graph, producing pictures of malnourished people, or explaining normal caloric needs are useless. I feel powerless to help. The things I wanted to say would only increase Meg's resistance to therapy.

It's a strange thing for a person to feel so hostile toward his or her own body. When Meg looked in the mirror, she saw an overweight person. "I am so fat, " she later said to me. In his memoir *A Leg to Stand On*, neurologist Oliver Sacks described estrangement from his own leg, which he injured in a freak accident with a wild ox. Similarly, some patients after a stroke have the bizarre sensation that a part of their body (like the right leg) is alien. They sometimes try to throw the "foreign" leg out of their beds, and to their surprise, drag themselves behind. Now, an entire diagnostic category—"body dysmorphic disordered"—describes individuals obsessed with the perceived ugly, or alien, appearance of their hands, noses, or other features, to the point where they stand in front of mirrors for hours, disgusted with themselves.

I explained the plan to Meg, "We're worried that your poor nutrition places you in serious danger. You'll be admitted to the hospital for a few days, and a special dietician will work with you to restore your health. This means gaining weight, but the weight will be lean weight and not fat. Your meals and bathroom visits will be supervised by a nurse or orderly." We talked a little longer. Meg and her parents had few questions, since they'd all been through this before. I wheeled Meg upstairs to the hospital wing used primarily for patients with eating disorders.

Meg lay down in her bed, stared out the window, and rebuffed my attempts at conversation. I left. Soon afterward, the dietician, Cassie Sanchez, performed measurements of Meg's body and created a detailed nutritional plan. Meg would eat increasing amounts of food daily until a target was reached. Additionally, she would be weighed daily to assess her progress.

Feeding an anorexic patient is a delicate task. In the 1940s, concentration camp survivors and prisoners of war suddenly fed after prolonged starvation developed acute swelling, heart failure, and, rarely, coma. This so-called refeeding syndrome was duplicated when American volunteers in the 1940s fasted for several weeks and then began eating. The symptoms were traced to accumulated deficiencies of certain vitamins and electrolytes. Today, emaciated people—whether hunger strikers, famine victims, or cancer patients—are always fed in a graduated manner and receive special vitamin supplements.

Meg's dinner included bread, broth, mashed potatoes, and a supplemental milkshake called Ensure. I sat in a chair to supervise her eating. It was a pitiful sight. Meg brought a spoonful of broth to her lips, began crying, and then pulled it away. When she finally mustered it into her mouth, she gagged and spit it out. The next spoonful got coughed out the same way. "I can't do it," she said, and put down her utensil.

The dietician's orders were very clear, I explained. I told Meg, "I'm sorry it's hard for you, but if you can't eat it by mouth, we'll have to put a tube through your nose and into your stomach to feed you." Called nasogastric feeding, this is a last resort for severe anorexics who won't eat. Meg tried a few more spoonfuls, with no result. "I just can't do it," she said. I called for the nurse.

Meg's nurse arrived in the room carrying a long, silicone nasogastric tube. It was the diameter of a pencil, but to Meg it must have seemed as wide as a garden hose. Experienced in the care of recalcitrant anorexics, Meg's nurse was very dramatic. In front of Meg, she unwrapped the tubing with coldly calculated care. She brandished the tubing, lubricated it with a dollop of oil, and sized up Meg's nose. "We're going to stick this up your nostril, and pass it down your esophagus into the stomach. It's fairly uncomfortable," she said, and paused for an interminable minute to inspect the tube. "Using it, we'll pass a liquefied meal directly into your gut," she continued, looking at Meg's belly.

"Let me try again," said Meg, shaken. Though she still gagged, Meg consumed her dinner within fifteen minutes. I congratulated her and left the room. Outside, Meg's nurse winked at me.

In the morning, the nurse asked Meg to remove her baggy clothing and step on a scale. She had gained an appropriate amount. The nurse sent a routine urine test and soon called me. "The urine's too dilute," she said. Despite having supervised meals and bathroom visits, Meg somehow had drunk a lot of water to artificially increase her weight. I told Meg that I knew she'd broken her restriction, and that a "one-to-one sitter," or an orderly who sat next to her at all times, was now necessary to protect her health.

The resourcefulness of anorexic patients is remarkable. To enhance their apparent weight, some place weights in their underwear, drink loads of water, or try various acrobatic maneuvers to press down harder on the scale. If they can't fool the scale, some sneak laxatives to purge their bodies or thyroid hormone to increase their metabolism after being weighed. Others find ways to exercise covertly by, for example, cycling their legs in bed for hours at night.

Under renewed scrutiny, Meg began gaining weight consistently. No further threats of nasogastric feeding were necessary. From school, teachers passed along assignments, and Meg worked diligently on her homework while sitting up in her hospital bed. The intensity she devoted to her schoolwork was telling.

Meg was an enigma. It's unlikely that her driving motivation was merely a desire to be seen as beautiful. While doing her schoolwork, Meg kept her pencil razor sharp, rotating it in a plastic sharpener after making each mark on a paper. She arranged her books exactly the same way every day and adjusted their angles periodically. While Meg simply could be seen as an organized person, I thought these behaviors exposed the crux of her anorexia: a desire for control.

A proposed—though controversial—risk factor for anorexia is an "enmeshed" family, in which children are overprotected and controlled by parents. For these children, who feel pressure to individuate themselves, exercising absolute control over the instinct to eat is empowering. Anorexia generally begins with simple dieting, which somehow, on being successful and reinforced by praise from parents or peers, develops into ritualized self-denial. One source described anorexia as "a shouting and unrelenting 'No,' which extends to every area of living, though most conspicuous in the food refusal." Just as certain individuals may abstain from sex for religious reasons, an anorexic patient rejects food to demonstrate mastery over one's primal drives. In addition, anorexics find a measure of control over one's family: no one, not even a child's parents, can really *make* the child eat.

But here's the paradox: the more the child tries to empower herself by not eating, the more she infantalizes herself. When Meg's parents visited her, she talked in a singsong voice instead of her usual tone. Now hospitalized, Meg seemed even more reliant on her parents. She'd call her mother and father twice a day to ask about her siblings, laughing one minute but castigating them for some perceived slight the next. Though sixteen years old, Meg had an elfin, childlike appearance since she was so small. She grew an infant's lanugo hair over her body. Like many malnourished women, she no longer menstruated. In the words of an expert on eating disorders, rather than becoming independent, anorexic patients "seem to be retreating further into childhood."

The cousin illness to anorexia nervosa is bulimia nervosa, or, literally, "ox hunger." While anorexia is characterized by extreme self-discipline, bulimia's hallmark is impulsivity. Like anorexics, bulimics are almost always women, but are usually of normal weight or slightly overweight. Bulimics may starve themselves for a few meals, but then engage in spectacular eating binges of up to 50,000 calories in a day—the amount a normal person eats in a month. Seized by guilt, the patient then vomits, fasts, or exercises until the next binge, which generally occurs about twice weekly.

Bulimia's psychopathology is distinct from anorexia's. Bulimia is best understood as a defective Pavlovian response: the presence of food induces uncontrollable desire, which isn't sated by eating normal amounts. Like rolling a snowball down a mountain, eating a small amount of a forbidden food—like ice cream—triggers an avalanche. One bulimic said, "I go on eating after I've satisfied [normal] hunger. I want to keep on eating until I feel full—it's the final limit. You can then eat no more."

Meg, on the other hand, just wanted to be thinner. When Meg vomited after meals, she wasn't feeling guilty from bingeing, but secretly purging meals in her endless quest to lose weight. With painstaking supervision in the hospital, Meg finally gained weight and ate her meals for four days straight. She was almost in remission. We prepared her discharge to a rehabilitation facility.

While I had temporarily helped stabilize Meg's weight, her long-term prognosis was unchanged. There is little evidence that any treatment—antidepressants, talk therapy, or residential programs in specialized centers—affects the course of the illness. A shocking number, about one in ten, eventually dies of starvation or other consequences of anorexia. Of the survivors, one in three retains anorexic behavior throughout her life.

Still, residential programs briefly can take pressure off a family by offering a middle ground between hospital and home. These "step-down" programs usually require admission for a few days or weeks. I contacted the psychiatrist on call, a Colombian woman named Luz Miraflores, to find a good center for Meg. Luz arrived, tied back her waist-length chestnut hair, and started working the phones. Her energy was dazzling. While much glory goes to doctors who perform dramatic resuscitations, cutting-edge research

for cancer cures, or cardiac transplants, unsung heroes like Luz
work in the background, using telephones instead of scalpels or
microscopes. Finding a good treatment center for a mentally ill
child is an exhausting ordeal; Luz routinely spent four hours calling
center after center for a depressed or anorexic child.

I went to lunch and returned. Luz was still in her chair, but she
was smiling. "I found one," she said. I wandered over to Meg's room
and told her the news.

"What time can I go?" asked Meg. "Maybe this afternoon, " I said,
and glanced at my watch. The date stood out, and I realized it was
my birthday.

Today was also Janmashtami, the birthday of the Hindu god
Krishna. Like the lustful Greek god of wine, Dionysius, who attracted
beautiful women called *bacchae*, Krishna was followed by *gopi* milk-
maids wherever he went. Throughout India, many parades and fes-
tivals are held to honor him on his birthday. In Bombay, earthen
pots are hung by pulleys over streets, and revelers make human pyr-
amids to reach and break them open like piñatas. The roads are
thronged during Janmashtami, a sensuous holiday that celebrates
Krishna's worldly passions.

Sitting in the hospital room, Meg and I were oddly juxtaposed.
Meg made a religion of extreme asceticism and self-denial. Unlike
her, I shared the worldview of Krishna, which demands not sepa-
rateness from the earth but ardent immersion into it. At the same
time, Meg and I did have something in common: we each pursued
an idealized version of ourselves. I hoped her quest was doomed to
failure, just as strongly as I hoped mine would succeed.

I have to make a confession. In the preface, I wrote that this book's
aim was to share some principles of pediatric medicine. This knowledge might offer the reader comfort when children in their lives
were ill, and also increase one's happiness when they were well. The

idea was to appreciate complete children by breaking them down into their parts.

The truth is, I wrote the book because I felt occasionally that this medical awareness has the opposite effect on me. Some days, I'd feel as though I'm not seeing patients, but just lungs and hearts and brains and bones and skin and guts. I can't make the leap to seeing whole people. Instead, they're reduced to their constituent organs. "Have you seen the ear in room five yet?" a nurse in the clinic might ask me. "No," I'd answer, "I'm busy with the belly in room two."

So this book is also about my quest to learn humanity. While writing about each organ, I thought about the various children for whom I cared. I also thought a lot about my father. In my memories, I saw his nosebleed at breakfast stemmed by platelets and heard the hissing of his ever-present oxygen tank. Then I saw the letters he wrote to my mother, and imagined how he carried her to the car when her leg broke. I remembered how his heart stopped and I felt his pulse for the last time. And then I recalled how his ashes touched my face. These memories all came to me together. I often felt guilty about medicalizing my father, and I used to try segregating intrusive thoughts about his platelets clumping and cardiovascular physiology from emotions of attachment and grief. But this endeavor was futile and unimportant. Ultimately, there was never a need to separate these perspectives, and never a need for guilt. Through writing, I realized that a physician can be simultaneously aware of people's organs and emotions, their cells and lived experiences—that is, develop a Zen-like, complementary sense of individuals' pieces and their wholes.

My son was born just after noon one crisp October day, at the Navajo hospital where I worked. Conceivably I could have been on call for my wife's delivery, but I'm thankful I wasn't. My roles as a son and doctor had already been blurred, and I was glad that my roles as a father and doctor weren't immediately so.

After our son's birth, my wife and I took turns feeding him overnight. He'd wake up and cry. On my nights, I'd arise and pick him up from his crib. He'd fuss, but I could console him by whispering into his ear. I'd pad downstairs to the kitchen and warm his bottle. Wide-eyed and alert, my son would see the bottle and open his mouth. He'd look so innocent, and I'd wonder what my father said to me when I was a baby. Yes, my son, we both might have said, I know you're hungry and need me. Listen to my voice as you absorb this nourishment from your gut and distribute it throughout your body, and know that, yes, I will always be here for you, I promise.

NOTES

PAGE   1. LUNGS

5   All of his internal organs began as microscopic pouches.   The
      standard textbook of human embryology is T. Sadler and J.
      Langman, *Langman's Medical Embryology*, 8th ed. (Baltimore:
      Lippincott, Williams & Wilkins, 2000).

5   Requiring oxygen just as humans do, the sea kelp must position
      every cell.   An evolutionary perspective on the respiratory sys-
      tem is found in William Keeton and James Gould, *Biological
      Science*, 6th ed. (New York: W. W. Norton, 1996).

6   Vance Tucker of Duke University has demonstrated.   V. Tucker,
      "Respiration during flight in birds," *Respiration Physiology* 14
      (1972): 75–82.

6   Biologist Lynn Margulis has hypothesized.   Lynn Margulis,
      *Symbiosis and Cell Evolution: Microbial Communities in the Archean and
      Proterozoic Eons*, 2d ed. (New York: W. H. Freeman & Co., 1992).

7   the misogynist term "hysteria" is derived from the Greek *hys-
      terikos*, or uterus.   *The American Heritage Dictionary of the English
      Language*, 4th ed. (Boston: Houghton Mifflin, 2000).

12   foods not recommended by the American Academy of Pediatrics for any toddler.   American Academy of Pediatrics, *Choking prevention and first aid for infants and children*, http://www.aap.org/family/choking.htm, accessed March 25, 2001.

13   Many years ago, the son of an artist named Sigmund Abeles was born.   Thomas Bolt, "Sigmund Abeles: The Max Drawings," *American Artist*, October 1987.

15   Adam was one of about 20,000 to 30,000 infants born yearly in the United States with immature lungs.   W. Oh and L. Stern, "Respiratory Diseases of the Newborn," in *Neonatal Medicine*, ed. L. Stern and P. Vert (New York: Masson Publishing, 1987).

15   Mary Ellen Avery, a pediatrician at Children's Hospital in Boston, discovered.   Avery wrote a fascinating lay account of her work in M. E. Avery, N. S. Wang, and H. W. Taeusch, "The lung of the newborn infant," *Scientific American* 228.4 (1973).

15   G. C. Liggins and R. N. Howie discovered that steroids injected into mothers.   G. C. Liggins and R. N. Howie, "A controlled trial of antepartum glucocorticoid treatment for prevention of the respiratory distress syndrome in premature infants," *Pediatrics* 50.4 (1972): 515–25.

15   In 1980, a group of Japanese pediatricians led by T. Fujiwara successfully took surfactant purified from cow lungs.   T. Fujiwara et al., "Artificial surfactant therapy in hyaline-membrane disease," *Lancet* 1.8159 (1980): 55–59.

19   The disease affects about one in twenty-five hundred white Americans.   C. Ruzal-Shapiro, "Cystic fibrosis: an overview," *Radiologic Clinics of North America* 36.1 (1998): 143–61.

19   Only about a quarter of these patients survives to adulthood, and less than one in ten lives past the age of thirty.   R. C. Boucher, "Cystic fibrosis," in *Harrison's Textbook of Internal Medicine*, ed. A. S. Fauci et al. (New York: McGraw-Hill, 1998).

19   In 1990, an international collaboration among biochemists discovered the cause of cystic fibrosis.   B. Kerem et al., "Identification of the cystic fibrosis gene: genetic analysis," *Science* 245.4922 (1989): 1073–80.

23   the faulty channel of CF may have protected generations of
      people from *Salmonella* infections.   G. B. Pier et al., "Salmonella
      typhi uses CFTR to enter intestinal epithelial cells," *Nature*
      393.6680 (1998): 79–82.

31   asthma is more prevalent (by 20 percent) among the urban
      poor . . . It is also more severe.   E. N. Grant, R. Wagner, and
      K. Weiss, "Observations on the emerging patterns of asthma in
      our society," *Journal of Allergy and Clinical Immunology* 104.2, pt. 2
      (1999): S1–9.

2. HEARTS

35   William Harvey, a sixteenth-century Oxford anatomist, exam-
      ined.   William Harvey and Geoffrey Keynes, *The Anatomical
      Exercises: De Motu Cordis and De Circulatione Sanguinis,* in English
      translation (New York: Dover Publications, 1995).

36   estimated to be almost one hundred thousand kilometers.
      Barry Zaret, Marvin Moser, and Lawrence Cohen, *Yale University
      School of Medicine Heart Book* (1992). Available at http://www.
      med.yale.edu/library/heartbk/.

38   About ninety-nine times out of a hundred, the folding works
      perfectly.   Richard E. Behrman, Robert Kliegman, and Hal B.
      Jenson, *Nelson Textbook of Pediatrics,* 16th ed. (Philadelphia: W. B.
      Saunders, 2000).

39   A child's heart is the end product of millions of years of evolu-
      tion.   The comparative anatomy of human and animal hearts
      is described in William T. Keeton, James L. Gould, and Carol
      Grant Gould, *Biological Science,* 4th ed. (New York: W. W. Norton,
      1986).

39   The neurologist Oliver Sacks writes that the joy of doctoring.
      Oliver W. Sacks, *The Man Who Mistook His Wife for a Hat and Other
      Clinical Tales* (New York: Summit Books, 1985).

40   In the vast majority of children, turbulent flow is a normal
      sound associated with a growing, healthy heart.   A. N. Pelech,
      "The cardiac murmur. When to refer?" *Pediatric Clinics of North
      America* 45.1 (1998): 107–22.

40   in his classic treatise *The Art and Science of Bedside Diagnosis*, Joseph Sapira offers the following advice.   Joseph Sapira, *The Art and Science of Bedside Diagnosis* (Baltimore: Williams & Wilkins, 1990).

41   she compensated by using her fingers to *feel* the sounds.   Sherwin B. Nuland, *Doctors: The Biography of Medicine* (New York: Knopf, 1988).

43   What we were performing had first been done in.   R. L. Mueller and T. A. Sanborn, "The history of interventional cardiology: cardiac catheterization, angioplasty, and related interventions," *American Heart Journal* 129.1 (1995): 146–72.

46   Medical historian Sherwin Nuland calls him "the greatest surgical scholar our country has ever produced."   Sherwin B. Nuland, *Doctors: The Biography of Medicine*, cited above.

47   In the epic Hindu poem *Mahabharata*.   William Buck and Shirley Triest, *Mahabharata* (Berkeley: University of California Press, 2000).

48   Samuel Shem, in his not-so-fictional best-seller *The House of God*.   Samuel Shem, *The House of God* (New York: R. Marek Publishers, 1978).

48   about sixty Americans per year die of tetanus.   Russell L. Cecil and Lee Goldman, *Cecil Textbook of Medicine*, 21st ed. (Philadelphia: W. B. Saunders, 2000).

50   In 1887, an enterprising surgeon named Langenbuch noted.   The early history of resuscitation is nicely reviewed in P. Juvin and J. M. Desmonts, "Cardiac massage: a method rescued from oblivion," *Anesthesiology* 89.3 (1998): 771–76.

50   In 1960, a landmark study by Kouwenhoven.   W. B. Kouwenhoven, J. R. Jude, and G. G. Knickerbocker, "Closed-chest cardiac massage," *Journal of the American Medical Association* 173 (1960): 1064–67.

51   one technique, active compression-decompression CPR, was developed after a man successfully resuscitated a family member with a household toilet plunger.   K. G. Lurie, C. Lindo, and J. Chin, "CPR: the P stands for plumber's helper," *Journal of the American Medical Association* 264.13 (1990): 1661.

56   Cardiac arrest patients have a 10 to 20 percent survival rate.   M. C. Thel and C. M. O'Connor, "Cardiopulmonary resuscitation: historical perspective to recent investigations," *American Heart Journal* 137.1 (1999): 39–48.

56   on television, cardiac arrest patients have a 75 percent rate of survival.   S. J. Diem, J. D. Lantos, and J. A. Tulsky, "Cardiopulmonary resuscitation on television," *New England Journal of Medicine* 334.24 (1996): 1578–82.

56   paramedical personnel successfully intubated children only half the time, and secured intravenous access only a third of the time. V. R. Kumar, D. T. Bachman, and R. T. Kiskaddon, "Children and adults in cardiopulmonary arrest: are advanced life support guidelines followed in the prehospital setting?" *Annals of Emergency Medicine* 29.6 (1997): 743–47.

3. BLOOD

61   In an 1882 article in the British medical journal *Lancet*, Bizzozero suggested.   M. U. Dianzani, "Bizzozero and the discovery of platelets," *American Journal of Nephrology* 14.4-6 (1994): 330–36.

61   In 1926, scientists at the University of Montreal confirmed his findings.   H. E. Burk and J. Tait, "Blood coagulation as by intravenous injection of tissue extract," *Quarterly Journal of Experimental Physiology* 16 (1925): 111–27.

62   one Talmudic reference to infant blood loss reads.   The full text of Yebamot 64b is found in Jacob Neusner, *Yebamot: Chicago Studies in the History of Judaism* (Chicago: University of Chicago Press, 1987).

63   In this manner, writes journalist Douglas Starr.   A fascinating account of Lambert's work can be found in Douglas P. Starr, *Blood: An Epic History of Medicine and Commerce* (New York: Alfred A. Knopf, 1998).

63   The twin discoveries of the ABO blood groups by Karl Landsteiner and citrate preservative by Richard Lewisohn.   K. Landsteiner, "Ueber agglutinationsersheinungen normalen menschlichen Blutes," *Wiener Klinische Wochenschrift* 14 (1901): 1132–34, and R.

Lewisohn, "The development of the technique of blood transfusion since 1907," *Archives of Mt. Sinai Medical Center* 10 (1944): 605–22.

64   the risk of acquiring viral hepatitis, HIV, or another infection . . . studies have shown that the risk of infection from related donors.   Harvey Klein, "Blood groups and blood transfusion," *Harrison's Principles of Internal Medicine*, ed. K. J. Isselbacher et. al. (New York: McGraw-Hill, 1994).

65   In 1929, the German biologist Henrik Dam found that chickens. Dam's discovery is detailed in his 1943 Nobel lecture (available at http://www.nobel.se/medicine/laureates/1943/dam-lecture.pdf) and in Henrik Dam, "Medical aspects of vitamin K," *Lancet* 63 (1943): 353.

66   Soon afterward Karl Link of the University of Wisconsin synthesized a derivative of dicumarol.   Wisconsin Alumni Research Foundation, *History of WARF*, http://www.wisc.edu/uir/warf.html, accessed February 18, 2002.

67   A recent report . . . found that almost 42 percent of Americans use herbal or dietary supplements and visit alternative practitioners, at an expense of $27 billion per year.   D. M. Eisenberg et al., "Unconventional medicine in the United States. Prevalence, costs, and patterns of use," *New England Journal of Medicine* 328.4 (1993): 246–52.

67   But as Marcia Angell and Jerome Kassirer of the *New England Journal of Medicine* point out.   M. Angell and J. P. Kassirer, "Alternative medicine—the risks of untested and unregulated remedies," *New England Journal of Medicine* 339.12 (1998): 839–41.

68   In an effort to frame this debate more constructively, the *Journal of the American Medical Association* editorialized in 1998.   P. B. Fontanarosa and G. D. Lundberg, "Alternative medicine meets science," *Journal of the American Medical Association* 280.18 (1998): 1618–19.

69   Bestselling author Dr. Andrew Weil writes.   A critique of Weil's work by a former editor of the *New England Journal of Medicine* is

A. Relman, "A Trip to Stonesville," *The New Republic*, 14 December 1998.

70   if we didn't possess such a wonderfully evolved method of oxygen delivery.   The evolution of red blood cells is described in "Oxygen-transporting proteins: myoglobin and hemoglobin," *Biochemistry*, ed. L. Stryer, 3d ed. (New York: W. H. Freeman & Co., 1988), 143–74.

72   "you know what the lady tells the slave? *Anything coming back to life hurts*."   Toni Morrison, *Beloved* (New York: Dutton Signet, 1988).

72   James Herrick, a Chicago doctor, discovered Monica's disease in 1904.   J. B. Herrick, "Peculiar elongated and sickle-shaped red blood corpuscles in a case of severe anemia," *Archives of Internal Medicine* 6 (1910): 517–21.

74   This problem intrigued biologist Anthony Allison.   A. C. Allison, "Sickle cells and evolution," *Scientific American* (1956): 87–94.

77   The notion . . . was tested by Samuel Charache at Johns Hopkins Hospital.   S. Charache et al., "Effect of hydroxyurea on the frequency of painful crises in sickle cell anemia," *New England Journal of Medicine* 332.20 (1995): 1317–22.

80   The cancer cells of a woman named Henrietta Lacks, who died in 1951, are so relentless.   Michael Gold, *A Conspiracy of Cells: One Woman's Immortal Legacy and the Medical Scandal It Caused* (Albany: State University of New York Press, 1986).

81   Perhaps the best-known leukemia patient at the time was Sadako Sasaki, a two-year-old.   Takayuki Ishii, *One Thousand Paper Cranes: The Story of Sadako and the Children's Peace Statue* (New York: Bantam Doubleday Dell Books for Young Readers, 2001).

81   At Yale University in the 1940s, Gilman noted this effect.   A. Gilman and F. S. Philips, "The biological actions and therapeutic applications of b-chloroethyl amines and sulfides," *Science* 103 (1946): 409.

81   Sidney Farber in Boston induced the first remission in pediatric leukemia.   S. Farber, L. K. Diamond, R. D. Mercer et. al., "Temporary remissions in acute leukemia in children produced by the

folic acid antagonist, 4-aminopteroyl-glutamic acid," *New England Journal of Medicine* 238 (1948): 787.

81   Based on these successes, the National Cancer Institute beginning in 1955 oversaw a remarkable program.   J. S. Driscoll, "The preclinical new drug research program of the National Cancer Institute," *Cancer Treatment Reports* 68 (1984): 63–76.

85   This wasn't literally true, as in the case of the "bubble boy" David Vetter.   Bruce Westbrook, "'Not a Comedy'—Family of 'Bubble Boy' Says Movie Insults Son's Legacy," *Houston Chronicle*, 15 August 2001.

87   Discovered in 1958 by the French researcher Jean Dausset, these proteins.   J. Dausset, "Iso-leuco-anticorps," *Acta Haematologica* 20 (1958): 156–66.

88   No national registry existed until 1977, when a ten-year-old girl named Laura Graves.   National Marrow Donor Program, *History of Stem Cell Transplants*, available at http://www.marrow. org/NMDP/history_stem_cell_transplants.html, accessed February 18, 2002.

89   In 1995, the parents of six-year-old Molly Nash were unable to find a match.   This remarkable case is described in Y. Verlinsky et al., "Preimplantation diagnosis for Fanconi anemia combined with HLA matching," *Journal of the American Medical Association* 285.24 (2001): 3130–33.

4. BONES

92   The most frequently injured joint of the body.   Keith Moore, *Clinically Oriented Anatomy*, 3d ed. (Baltimore: Williams & Wilkins, 1992).

95   the twenty-sixth day of development, half of the groove closes.   M. M. Iqbal, "Prevention of neural tube defects by periconceptional use of folic acid," *Pediatrics in Review* 21.2 (2000): 58–66.

96   Lucy Wills in 1931 had begun work that would eventually absolve.   L. Wills, "Treatment of 'pernicious anemia of pregnancy' and 'tropical anemia' with special reference to yeast extract as a curative agent," *British Medical Journal* 1.1059 (1931).

96   William Osler noted that.   W. Osler, "The severe anemias of pregnancy and the post-partum state," *British Medical Journal* 1 (1919): 1.

97   a biochemist at the University of Texas . . . a half-ton of spinach. H. K. Mitchell, E. E. Snell, and R. J. Williams, "The concentration of 'folic acid,'" *Journal of the American Chemical Society* 63 (1941): 2284.

97   an obstetrician reported that almost 70 percent of his patients who delivered children.   B. M. Hibbard, "The role of folic acid in pregnancy," *Journal of Obstetrics and Gynaecology of the British Commonwealth* 71 (1964): 529–42.

97   A large trial involving almost two thousand English women was prematurely ended.   Medical Research Council Vitamin Study Research Group, "Prevention of neural tube defects: Results of the Medical Research Council vitamin study," *Lancet* 338.8760 (1991): 131–37.

97   In the words of Robert Brent.   R. L. Brent, G. P. Oakley, Jr., and D. R. Mattison, "The unnecessary epidemic of folic acid–preventable spina bifida and anencephaly," *Pediatrics* 106.4 (2000): 825–27.

98   Recently, in South Carolina, a well-funded campaign.   R. E. Stevenson et al., "Decline in prevalence of neural tube defects in a high-risk region of the United States," *Pediatrics* 106.4 (2000): 677–83.

98   In 1996, the U.S. Food and Drug Administration ordered. Food and Drug Administration, U.S. Department of Health and Human Services, "Food standards: amendment of the standards of identity for enriched grain products to require addition of folic acid," *Federal Register* 61 (1996): 8781–807.

98   the proportion of women consuming enough folate.   American Academy of Pediatrics, "Folic acid for the prevention of neural tube defects," *Pediatrics* 104.2 (1999): 325–27.

98   folate is safe even in large amounts.   C. E. Butterworth, Jr., and T. Tamura, "Folic acid safety and toxicity: a brief review," *American Journal of Clinical Nutrition* 50.2 (1989): 353–58.

99   described in detail by James Gleick.   James Gleick, *Chaos: Making a New Science* (New York: Viking, 1987).

99   a surprise outbreak of an acute paralysis called Guillain-Barré. T. J. Safranek et al., "Reassessment of the association between Guillain-Barré syndrome and receipt of swine influenza vaccine in 1976–1977: Results of a two-state study." *American Journal of Epidemiology* 133.9 (1991): 940–51.

99   In a 1989 national survey of almost one thousand practicing blood specialists.   C. E. Butterworth, Jr., and T. Tamura, "Folic acid safety and toxicity: a brief review," cited above.

99   many nutritionists have pointed out that a strategy of adding *both* vitamin B_{12} and folate.   G. P. Oakley, Jr., "Let's increase folic acid fortification and include vitamin B-12," *American Journal of Clinical Nutrition* 65.6 (1997): 1889–90.

100   the first medical X ray taken in North America.   P. K. Spiegel, "The first clinical X ray made in America—100 years," *American Journal of Roentgenology* 164.1 (1995): 241–43.

102   Giovanni Monteggia, who described dislocations.   T. Laor, D. Jaramillo, and A. Oestreich, "Musculoskeletal System," in *Practical Pediatric Imaging: Radiology of Infants and Children*, ed. D. Kirks, 3d ed. (Philadelphia: Lippincott-Raven, 1998).

103   Before a child reaches one year of age every one of his 206 bones.   A. Rosenberg, "Bones, Joints, and Soft Tissue Tumors," in *Robbins' Pathologic Basis of Disease*, ed. Vinay Kumar, Stanley L. Robbins, and Ramzi S. Cotran, 6th ed. (Philadelphia: W. B. Saunders, 1999).

106   Mandl strategically placed his code team.   Kenneth Mandl, interview with author, 20 September 1999.

107   "I knew what that meant," she later said.   Court TV, televised trial of Louise Woodward, 5 October 1997.

108   In 1946, he published the abstruse-sounding.   J. Caffey, "Multiple fractures in long bones of infants suffering from chronic subdural hematoma," *American Journal of Roentgenology* 56 (1946): 163–73.

108   The dubious nature of these bleeds was described as early as A.D. 200.   Richard Krugman, *Public Health, Politics, and Child Protection:*

Can We Do Better in the Next Millennium? Grand Rounds lecture at Children's Hospital, Boston, 5 May 1999.

108   The first physician to study infant brain bleeds systematically, the nineteenth-century.   The early history of child abuse is discussed comprehensively by P. C. English and H. Grossman, "Radiology and the history of child abuse," *Pediatric Annals* 12 (1983): 870–74, and in passing by other articles in the same journal issue, which is devoted to child abuse.

109   he insisted that a radiologist "must stand his ground."   J. Caffey, "Some traumatic lesions in growing bones other than fractures and dislocations: clinical and radiological features," *British Journal of Radiology* 30 (1957): 225–38.

109   Frustrated, he once wrote.   Ibid.

110   defined the "battered child syndrome" in the *Journal of the American Medical Association.*   C. H. Kempe et al., "The battered-child syndrome," *Journal of the American Medical Association* 181.1 (1962): 105–12.

110   Frederic Silverman, who was Caffey's first trainee and protégé.   F. N. Silverman, "Unrecognized trauma in infants, the battered child syndrome, and the syndrome of Ambroise Tardieu. Rigler Lecture," *Radiology* 104.2 (1972): 337–53.

110   Paul Kleinman's classic textbook on child abuse.   Paul K. Kleinman, *Diagnostic Imaging of Child Abuse,* 2d ed. (St. Louis, Mo.: Mosby, 1998).

111   In 1873, for example, the Catholic missionary Etta Wheeler.   S. Lazoritz, "Child Abuse: An Historical Perspective," in *Child Abuse: A Medical Reference,* ed. S. Ludwig and A. Kornberg, 2d ed. (New York: Churchill Livingston, 1992), 85–90; S. Lazoritz, "Whatever happened to Mary Ellen," *Child Abuse and Neglect* 14 (1990): 143; and Lela B. Costin, Howard Jacob Karger, and David Stoesz, *The Politics of Child Abuse in America* (New York: Oxford University Press, 1996).

114   Newberger, who founded the CPT in 1970.   Eli Newberger, personal interviews, e-mail communications, and telephone interviews with author, April–August 1999; and E. Newberger, "The

Medicine of the Tuba," in *Doctors Afield*, ed. Mary G. McCrea Curnen, Howard M. Spiro, and Deborah St. James (New Haven: Yale University Press, 1999).

114   Described originally in the British medical journal *Lancet* in 1977 as the "hinterland."   R. Meadow, "Munchausen syndrome by proxy: the hinterland of child abuse," *Lancet* 2.8033 (1977): 343–45.

115   Joseph Madsen, a stocky senior neurosurgeon.   Joseph Madsen, interview with author, July 1999.

117   Byrne called Mandl, who told him.   William Byrne, telephone interview with author, 16 November 1999.

118   One British tabloid pontificated, "American justice. . . ."   Aileen McCabe, "British media outraged by au pair verdict," *Gazette*, 2 November 1997.

118   the London *Guardian* commented.   Sarah Lyall, "The nation: an American jury shocks Britain," *New York Times*, 2 November 1997.

119   Alan Dershowitz wondered on CNN's *Larry King Live*.   Alan Dershowitz, televised interview on *Larry King Live* (CNN), 30 October 1997. Transcript available at http://www.cnn.com/transcripts/lkl.html, accessed December 1998.

119   two pediatricians from Cleveland County in Leeds, England.   C. J. Hobbs and J. M. Wynne, "Buggery in childhood—a common syndrome of child abuse," *Lancet* 2.8510 (1986): 792–96.

119   years later the *Sunday Telegraph* bemoaned.   Anthea Hall, "Cleveland doctors 'lose public trust,'" *Sunday Telegraph* (London), 25 September 1988.

119   Americans witnessed the retraction of entire "diseases."   Joan Acocella, "The politics of hysteria," *The New Yorker*, 6 April 1998; 64–79.

119   one Boston laborer told *USA Today*.   John Larrabee, "Irish immigrants rallying to cause of British au pair," *USA Today*, 6 November 1997.

119   Woodward "was given too much responsibility."   Sherryl

Connelly, "Feel sorry for the parents," *New York Daily News*, 11 November 1997.

119 "She is guilty of manslaughter," referring not to Woodward. Ellen Goodman, "Who gets blamed next for Matthew's death? Working mother, of course," *Boston Globe*, 26 October 1997.

120 the best pediatric facility in the country yearly for over a decade "America's Best Hospitals," *U.S. News and World Report*, 23 July 2001.

120 Leone sat at his desk.   Gerard Leone, Jr., interview with author, 25 August 1999.

121 On October 7, 1997, Leone said.   The trial was carried unedited on Court TV, from which direct quotes and chronology information are derived. For brevity's sake, references regarding events from the trial will not be individually cited. A substantial archive of information regarding the Woodward trial, including audio and video clips, is also available at http://www.courttv.com/casefiles/nanny/nanny.html. Some information is also taken from various articles from the *Boston Globe* during the trial.

122 Conversely, they are deadly for the same reasons when retracted. Over the following two days, Scheck repeated the analogy to neurosurgeon Joseph Madsen, radiologist Patrick Barnes, and Feigin, who each retreated from it without offering a clearer alternative. Under direct cross-examination from Scheck, Madsen admitted that it was misleading and that he had only made the comparison "in response to a very specific question" during grand jury testimony. When asked if he could support Leone's claim that Matthew had been shaken for "about a minute," Barnes responded that he thought Matthew had been traumatized but couldn't estimate a time (roughly "how many shakes and how many impacts") that the child suffered.

On the fourth day of testimony, Gerald Feigin also explained that his autopsy findings didn't support Newberger's prior estimate to the grand jury that Matthew had been shaken violently for about a minute. "It would have been physically difficult to shake a twenty-two-pound baby violently for that amount of time," he said. He then confessed that he was mistaken when he had told a grand jury that Matthew's head injury was the "equivalent of one suffered from a fifteen-foot fall onto a hard surface." In fact, he said, the baby's skull fracture could have resulted under some circumstances from a fall of a few feet.

123 In her book *Science on Trial*, Marcia Angell.   Marcia Angell, *Science on Trial : The Clash of Medical Evidence and the Law in the Breast Implant Case* (New York: W. W. Norton, 1996).

123 In a *Wall Street Journal* commentary, Harvey Silverglate.   Harvey Silverglate, "Science and the Au Pair Trial," *Wall Street Journal*, 11 November 1997.

123 He later told me, "once the first doctor."   Harvey Silverglate, e-mail communication with author, 6 October 1999.

124 he later called the case "the single most agonizing."   "Mass Lawyer Story: Harvey A. Silverglate," *Massachusetts Lawyers Weekly*, 28 December 1998, 27.

125 he condemned as an opportunistic defensive ploy.   J. Godwin Greenfield and J. Hume Adams, *Greenfield's Neuropathology*, 5th ed. (New York: Oxford University Press, 1992).

126 by a widely cited 1992 study by Ann-Christine Duhaime.   A. C. Duhaime et al., "Head injury in very young children: mechanisms, injury types, and ophthalmologic findings in 100 hospitalized patients younger than 2 years of age," *Pediatrics* 90.2, pt. 1 (1992): 179–85.

127 Thibault, a scientific purist who abhors any speculation, told me. Lawrence Thibault, telephone interview with author, 3 November 1999.

127 On October 28, closing arguments were made.   "Excerpts of Woodward closing arguments," *Boston Globe*, 29 October 1997.

129 Zobel has the bearing of a patrician   Hiller Zobel, telephone interviews with author, 3 and 10 November 1999.

129 The *Boston Globe* praised Zobel's judicial wisdom.   "Judge Zobel's justice," *Boston Globe*, 11 November 1997.

129 The *New York Times* joined the adulation.   "Justice restored," *New York Times*, 11 November 1997.

130 was reproached by some Newton residents in *Time*.   David Sapsted, "Hate mail for Eappens as au pair awaits fate," *Daily Telegraph* (London), 10 November 1997; Terry McCarthy, "A Stunning Verdict," *Time*, 10 November 1997.

130 *Pediatrics* published a letter signed by forty-seven academic pediatricians.   D. L. Chadwick et al., "Shaken baby syndrome—a forensic pediatric response," *Pediatrics* 101.2 (1998): 321–23.

130 The *New England Journal of Medicine* then published an educational article.   A. C. Duhaime et al., "Nonaccidental head injury in infants—the 'shaken-baby syndrome,'" *New England Journal of Medicine* 338.25 (1998): 1822–29.

130 Harvey Silverglate suggested that Matthew may have been injured by his two-year-old brother.   "Mass Lawyer Story: Harvey A. Silverglate," cited above.

130 Jan Leestma, at the request of a defense lawyer, handed.   Don Aucoin and Shelley Murphy, "Defense shared Eappen tissue," *Boston Globe*, 10 March 1999; Don Aucoin, "Wallace says show seeks truth before ratings," *Boston Globe*, 9 March 1999.

130 After shopping around the tissues to several specialists nationwide, she made contact with Floyd Gilles.   The previous February, defense attorney Elaine Whitfield-Sharp consulted thirty-five medical experts about the same samples, including Gilles and Nelson, without hearing a similar story. In a bizarre twist, she was stopped for drunk driving some months later, and told arresting officer Randy Cipoletta that she was pushed to drink and drive from the stress of working for a guilty client, Louise Woodward.

132 Kathleen McCarthy, the department manager.   Kathleen McCarthy, interview with author, 26 May 1999.

132 In his book on multiple personality disorder, *Multiple Identities and False Memories*.   Nicholas P. Spanos, *Multiple Identities and False Memories: A Sociocognitive Perspective* (Washington, D.C.: American Psychological Association, 1996).

133 In his 1906 short story "Sleepy-Eye," Anton Chekhov.   Anton Chekhov, "Sleepy-Eye," *Cosmopolitan*, May 1906: 151–56.

133   child death review teams in Colorado and Oregon.   Oregon
       Department of Human Services, *Child Death in Oregon, 1998:
       Oregon Child Fatality Review Team Annual Report* (Portland: Oregon
       Health Division, 1999); Richard Krugman, telephone interview
       with author, 30 May 1999.

133   Scores of psychological studies suggest that physical.   M. T.
       Stein and E. L. Perrin, "Guidance for effective discipline," *Pediatrics*
       101.4, pt. 1 (1998): 723–28.

134   about one-quarter of American parents hit their kids.   Murray
       A. Straus and Denise A. Donnelly, *Beating the Devil Out of Them:
       Corporal Punishment in American Families and Its Effects on Children*
       (New Brunswick, N.J.: Transaction, 2001).

134   The Elmira program created by David Olds in Denver.   J. Ecken-
       rode et al., "Child maltreatment and the early onset of problem
       behaviors: Can a program of nurse home visitation break the
       link?," *Development and Psychopathology* 13.4 (2001): 873–90.

5. BRAINS

137   A worm called *Taenia solium* had caused the lesions on the pig's
       tongue.   A comprehensive review about cysticercosis infec-
       tions is H. H. Garcia and O. H. Del Brutto, "Taenia solium cys-
       ticercosis," *Infectious Disease Clinics of North America* 14.1 (2000):
       97–119.

139   In the words of economist Thomas Schelling, a free society is
       "an ecology of micromotives."   Thomas Schelling, "An ecology
       of micromotives," *The Corporate Society*, ed. Robin L. Marris
       (London: MacMillan, 1974).

139   About one in five Americans has such an event at some time.
       Ilo Leppik, *Contemporary Diagnosis and Management of the Patient
       with Epilepsy*, 3d ed. (Newtown, Pa.: Associates in Medical Mar-
       keting Company, 1997).

139   the Greek for breeze is *aura*.   *The American Heritage Dictionary of
       the English Language*, 4th ed. (Boston: Houghton Mifflin, 2000).

139   Michael Crichton's bestseller *The Terminal Man*.   Michael Crich-
       ton, *The Terminal Man* (New York: Knopf, 1972).

140   In 1987, a Canadian outbreak of prolonged seizures.   T. M. Perl et al., "An outbreak of toxic encephalopathy caused by eating mussels contaminated with domoic acid," *New England Journal of Medicine* 322.25 (1990): 1775–80.

141   Phenytoin is a type of barbiturate or sedative developed after 1912.   W. J. Friedlander, "Putnam, Merritt, and the discovery of Dilantin," *Epilepsia* 27, suppl. 3 (1986): S1–20.

141   The story of valproic acid, another key antiepileptic drug.   S. L. McElroy and P. E. Keck, "Anti-epileptic drugs," in *Textbook of Psychopharmacology*, ed. A. Schatzberg and C. B. Nemeroff (Washington, D.C.: American Psychiatric Press, 1995) 351–75.

143   On December 16, 1997, an episode of the cartoon show *Pokémon*. B. Radford and R. Bartholomew, "Pokémon contagion: photosensitive epilepsy or mass psychogenic illness?," *Southern Medical Journal* 94.2 (2001): 197–204, and T. Hayashi et al., "Pocket Monsters, a popular television cartoon, attacks Japanese children," *Annals of Neurology* 44.3 (1998): 427–28.

144   But in 1990, a small epidemic of brain cysticercosis occurred in an Orthodox Jewish community.   P. M. Schantz et al., "Neurocysticercosis in an Orthodox Jewish community in New York City," *New England Journal of Medicine* 327.10 (1992): 692–95.

145   The first modern public health intervention took place in 1854. S. Tanihara et al., "Snow on cholera," *Journal of Epidemiology* 8.4 (1998): 185–94.

145   in fact, the last naturally occurring case in the entire Western Hemisphere occurred in Peru in 1991.   F. C. Robbins, "Eradication of polio in the Americas," *Journal of the American Medical Association* 270.15 (1993): 1857–59.

146   In certain Peruvian areas of endemic infection, newborn "sentinel" pigs are placed.   A. E. Gonzalez et al., "Use of sentinel pigs to monitor environmental Taenia solium contamination," *American Journal of Tropical Medicine and Hygiene* 51.6 (1994): 847–50.

147   The Navajo refer to themselves as the Diné.   Translations and background information on the Navajo are from Raymond F.

Locke, *The Book of the Navajo*, 5th ed. (Los Angeles: Mankind Publishing Co., 1992). Statistics about Gallup crime are from Raymond Daw and Herb Moser, "The Bridges of McKinley County: Building Rural Recovery Coalitions," *Treating Alcohol and Other Drug Abusers in Rural and Frontier Areas* (1995), Department of Health and Human Services Publication No. (SMA) 95-3054.

147   In his novel *The Quincunx*, Charles Palliser writes.   Charles Palliser, *The Quincunx* (New York: Ballantine Books, 1990).

149   the brain has a functional organization first outlined by Wilder Penfield.   W. Feindel, "Wilder Penfield (1891–1976): The man and his work," *Neurosurgery* 1.2 (1977): 93–100.

150   In 1869, Douglas Argyll Robertson noticed.   C. C. Dacso and D. L. Bortz, "Significance of the Argyll Robertson pupil in clinical medicine," *American Journal of Medicine* 86.2 (1989): 199–202.

151   Marcia Herman-Giddens found.   M. E. Herman-Giddens et al., "Secondary sexual characteristics and menses in young girls seen in office practice: a study from the Pediatric Research in Office Settings network," *Pediatrics* 99.4 (1997): 505–12.

151   Several famous people have had this condition.   Chris Dufresne, "Requiem for a giant," *Los Angeles Times*, 23 February 1993; "Rondo Hatton in jungle captive," *Irish Times*, 7 April 2001; and Dennis McLellan, "Shedding light on a rare disease," *Los Angeles Times*, 27 December 1992.

151   Ben-Gurion University neurologist Vladimir Berginer believes that the biblical giant Goliath.   V. M. Berginer, "Neurological aspects of the David-Goliath battle: restriction in the giant's visual field," *Israel Medical Association Journal* 2.9 (2000): 725–27.

152   the same words that J. Robert Oppenheimer did upon seeing the detonation of the world's first atomic weapon.   John Bartlett and Justin Kaplan, *Familiar Quotations*, 16th ed. (Boston: Little, Brown, 1992).

154   in the 1980's, a careless drug dealer in California caused an outbreak of Parkinson's disease.   P. A. Ballard, J. W. Tetrud, and

J. W. Langston, "Permanent human parkinsonism due to 1-methyl-4-phenyl-1,2,3,6- tetrahydropyridine (MPTP): seven cases," *Neurology* 35.7 (1985): 949–56.

155   a scene where Harry Potter's class learns to fight magical creatures called *boggarts.* J. K. Rowling, *Harry Potter and the Prisoner of Azkaban* (London: Bloomsbury, 1999).

157   In 1973, Congress passed the Rehabilitation Act, which includes Section 504.   A review of the laws regarding learning disabilities is Community Alliance for Special Education, *Special Education Rights and Responsibilities*, 8th ed. (San Francisco: CASE and PAI, 2000). An excerpt is available at http://www.pai-ca.org/pubs/504101.htm.

157   the Supreme Court in 1982 ruled in *Board of Education v. Rowley.* U.S. Supreme Court, *Hendrick Hudson District Board of Education v. Rowley*, 458 U.S. 176 (1982).

159   In 1993, I wrote a health survey administered by the Kentucky Department.   *Kentucky Health Interview and Examination Study 1993* (Frankfort, Ky.: World Wide Printing, 1995).

161   Psychologist Edwin Boring showed the tautological nature of these definitions in 1923.   Earl Hunt, "The role of intelligence in modern society," *American Scientist*, July–August 1995.

163   psychiatrist Charles Bradley decided to try a drug called Benzedrine.   C. Bradley, "The behavior of children receiving benzedrine," *American Journal of Psychiatry* 94 (1937): 577–85.

163   In Germany, L. Edeleano had synthesized the compound some fifty years earlier.   L. Edeleano, "Uber einige Derivate der Phenylmethacrylsaure und der Phenylisobuttersaure," *Berichte der deutschen chemischen Gesellschaft* 20 (1887): 616.

164   Drug Enforcement Administration production quotas for methylphenidate.   Drug Enforcement Administration, *Yearly Aggregate Production Quotas* (Washington, D.C.: Drug Enforcement Administration Office of Public Affairs, 1995).

164   In Maryland, which tracks statewide treatment statistics for children with ADHD.   D. J. Safer, J. M. Zito, and E. M. Fine, "Increased

methylphenidate usage for attention deficit disorder in the 1990s," *Pediatrics* 98.6, pt. 1 (1996): 1084–88.

164 the *Diagnostic and Statistical Manual of Mental Disorders* defines all currently known psychiatric disorders.   American Psychiatric Association and American Psychiatric Association Task Force on DSM-IV, *Diagnostic and Statistical Manual of Mental Disorders: DSM-IV*, 4th ed. (Washington, D.C.: American Psychiatric Association, 1994).

164 In the late 1980s, studies in the United States estimated that 6 to 7 percent of *all* children met this definition.   J. C. Anderson et al., "DSM-III disorders in preadolescent children: Prevalence in a large sample from the general population," *Archives of General Psychiatry* 44.1 (1987): 69–76.

164 When compared to normal children, those with ADHD are. S. L. Block, "Attention-deficit disorder: a paradigm for psychotropic medication intervention in pediatrics," *Pediatric Clinics of North America* 45.5 (1998): 1053–83.

164 the average visit where ADHD is diagnosed lasts only thirty-eight minutes and is billable at only one-tenth of our fee. Less than two-thirds of providers take the time.   L. Copeland et al., "Pediatricians' reported practices in the assessment and treatment of attention deficit disorders," *Journal of Developmental and Behavioral Pediatrics* 8.4 (1987): 191–97.

165 parent reports of their child's behavior in school were very different than teacher reports.   E. M. Mitsis et al., "Parent-teacher concordance for DSM-IV attention-deficit/hyperactivity disorder in a clinic-referred sample," *Journal of the American Academy of Child and Adolescent Psychiatry* 39.3 (2000): 308–13.

165 As recommended by the American Academy of Pediatrics in 2001, behavior therapy is an effective adjunct.   American Academy of Pediatrics, "Clinical practice guideline: treatment of the school-aged child with attention-deficit/hyperactivity disorder," *Pediatrics* 108.4 (2001): 1033–44.

165 In 1974, the allergist Ben Feingold claimed.   Ben F. Feingold, *Why Your Child Is Hyperactive* (New York: Random House, 1974).

166   Russel Barkley wrote.   R. A. Barkley, "A review of stimulant drug research with hyperactive children," *Journal of Child Psychology and Psychiatry* 18.2 (1977): 137–65.

6. SKIN

168   this skin-to-skin method of keeping an infant warm was developed at a Bogotá, Colombia, hospital.   G. F. Kirsten, N. J. Bergman, and F. M. Hann, "Kangaroo mother care in the nursery," *Pediatric Clinics of North America* 48.2 (2001): 443–52.

169   Though Heron of Alexandria had developed an instrument measuring thermal changes.   E. A. Dominguez, A. Bar-Sela, and D. M. Musher, "Adoption of thermometry into clinical practice in the United States," *Reviews of Infectious Diseases* 9.6 (1987): 1193–201.

169   With the benefit of Fahrenheit's device, Herman Boerhaave.   D. C. Smith, "The rise and fall of typhomalarial fever: Origins," *Journal of the History of Medicine and Allied Sciences* 37.2 (1982): 182–220.

169   This hypothesis led Carl Wunderlich in Germany to study comprehensively the distribution.   C. Wunderlich, *Das Verhalten der Eigenwärme in Krankheiten* (Leipzig, Germany: Otto Wogard, 1868).

169   the 1990 edition of *Stedman's Medical Dictionary* defines fever as "a bodily temperature above the normal of 98.6°F."   Thomas Stedman, *Stedman's Medical Dictionary*, 25th ed. (Baltimore: Williams & Wilkins, 1990).

169   average body temperature is actually closer to 98.2 degrees according to more recent studies.   P. A. Mackowiak, S. S. Wasserman, and M. M. Levine, "A critical appraisal of 98.6 degrees F, the upper limit of the normal body temperature, and other legacies of Carl Reinhold August Wunderlich," *Journal of the American Medical Association* 268.12 (1992): 1578–80.

172   First described in 1921 as an "ammoniacal scald," diaper rash occurs in about one in five infants.   E. L. Kazaks and A. T. Lane, "Diaper dermatitis," *Pediatric Clinics of North America* 47.4 (2000): 909–19.

172   As science journalist Malcolm Gladwell delicately points out. Malcolm Gladwell, "Smaller," *The New Yorker,* 26 November 2001.

174   Scores of studies looking at conference attendance . . . all recapitulate the same story.   W. R. Smith, "Evidence for the effectiveness of techniques to change physician behavior," *Chest* 118.2, suppl. (2000): 8S–17S.

174   In a publicized 1978 report, the U.S. Office of Technology Assessment concluded.   Office of Technology Assessment, *Assessing the Efficacy and Safety of Medical Technologies* (Washington, D.C.: Congress of the United States Office of Technology Asssesment, 1978).

175   only 40 percent of pediatric care is supported by high-quality data.   M. C. Rudolf et al., "A search for the evidence supporting community paediatric practice," *Archives of Disease in Childhood* 80.3 (1999): 257–61.

176   the antivenin itself carried a small risk of inducing a fatal allergic reaction.   G. R. Bond, "Snake, spider, and scorpion envenomation in North America," *Pediatrics in Review* 20.5 (1999): 147–50.

177   In the late 1960s, psychiatrist John Bowlby developed a framework called attachment theory.   J. Bowlby, *Attachment and Loss,* vol. 1 (London: Hogarth Press and the Institute of Psycho-Analysis, 1969).

178   As another psychologist later summarized, "The experience of security."   P. Fonagy, M. Target, and G. Gergely, "Attachment and borderline personality disorder: a theory and some evidence," *Psychiatry Clinics of North America* 23.1 (2000): 103–22.

178   In the 1970s, Mary Ainsworth developed a laboratory procedure called the "Strange Situation."   M. Ainsworth et al., *Patterns of Attachment: A Psychological Study of the Strange Situation* (Hillsdale, N.J.: Erlbaum, 1978).

179   three-quarters of people maintain the same attachment classification.   E. Waters et al., "From the strange situation to the adult attachment interview: a 20-year longitudinal study of attachment security in infancy and early adulthood." Conference pro-

ceedings, Society for Research in Child Development, Indianapolis, May 1995.

180   As a medical student he developed a novel method of repairing a pediatric heart defect and was the first student. Judah Folkman, "The discovery of angiogenesis inhibitors: a new class of drugs." Marine Biological Laboratories Friday Evening Lecture series, Woods Hole, Mass., 15 June 2001.

181   In 1988, Folkman received a call from Carl White of Denver. C. W. White et al., "Treatment of pulmonary hemangiomatosis with recombinant interferon alfa-2a," *New England Journal of Medicine* 320.18 (1989): 1197–200.

181   Folkman convened a larger study. R. A. Ezekowitz, J. B. Mulliken, and J. Folkman, "Interferon alfa-2a therapy for life-threatening hemangiomas of infancy," *New England Journal of Medicine* 326.22 (1992): 1456–63.

183   pediatricians recommend shielding the scar from prolonged sunlight and occasionally using vitamin E lotions. L. S. Baumann and J. Spencer, "The effects of topical vitamin E on the cosmetic appearance of scars," *Dermatologic Surgery* 25.4 (1999): 311–15, and K. L. Keller and N. A. Fenske, "Uses of vitamins A, C, and E and related compounds in dermatology: A review," *Journal of the American Academy of Dermatology* 39.4, pt. 1 (1998): 611–25.

184   derived from either the Old English *gican*, meaning itch, or the Old French word *chiche-pois*, meaning chickpea. J. H. Scott-Wilson, "Why 'chicken' pox?," *Lancet* 1.8074 (1978): 1152; C. Grose and T. I. Ng, "Intracellular synthesis of varicella-zoster virus," *Journal of Infectious Diseases* 166, suppl. 1 (1992): S7–12.

184   Until 1767, chickenpox and its deadlier imitator smallpox were not distinguished. J. E. Gordon, "Chickenpox: an epidemiological review," *American Journal of the Medical Sciences* 244 (1962): 362–89.

184   90 percent of all children younger than ten years have had chickenpox. Ninety-nine percent of adults have varicella antibodies. M. Wharton, "The epidemiology of varicella-zoster virus

infections," *Infectious Disease Clinics of North America* 10.3 (1996): 571–81.

184   parents often saw the illness as a child's rite of passage and had parties to disseminate the infection.   Evelyn Yap, "It's party time for parents who want kids to get chicken pox," *Straits Times*, 10 August 1996; Rashida Dhooma, "Rushing mother nature; docs frown on chicken pox 'parties,'" *Toronto Sun*, 28 August 1995.

185   The vaccine is traceable to a three-year-old Japanese boy.   M. Takahashi et al., "Live vaccine used to prevent the spread of varicella in children in hospital," *Lancet* 2.7892 (1974): 1288–90.

186   several vaccines, including Albert Sabin's celebrated polio vaccine, were cultivated using such cells.   Stanley A. Plotkin and Walter A. Orenstein, *Vaccines*, 3d ed. (Philadelphia: W. B. Saunders, 1999).

186   only one-third of American toddlers got the vaccine in 1998, and in some states only one in twenty did.   American Academy of Pediatrics, "Varicella vaccine update," *Pediatrics* 105.1, pt. 1 (2000): 136–41.

186   In a 1998 letter to the *New England Journal of Medicine*, two doctors wrote.   R. W. Spingarn and J. A. Benjamin, "Universal vaccination against varicella," *New England Journal of Medicine* 338.10 (1998): 683.

186   Similar opposition to vaccination existed during a 1901 epidemic of smallpox.   This episode is reviewed in M. R. Albert, K. G. Ostheimer, and J. G. Breman, "The last smallpox epidemic in Boston and the vaccination controversy, 1901–1903," *New England Journal of Medicine* 344.5 (2001): 375–79.

187   The resulting immunity from both easily lasts for twenty years. A. A. Gershon, "Live-attenuated varicella vaccine," *Infectious Disease Clinics of North America* 15.1 (2001): 65–81.

189   At Children's Hospital, the rate of bloodstream infections linked to chickenpox tripled.   A. Doctor, M. B. Harper, and G. R. Fleisher, "Group A beta-hemolytic streptococcal bacteremia: historical overview, changing incidence, and recent association with varicella," *Pediatrics* 96.3, pt. 1 (1995): 428–33.

189   In the early 1990s, varicella caused ten thousand hospitaliza-

tions per year and over one hundred deaths. S. A. Plotkin, "Varicella vaccine," *Pediatrics* 97.2 (1996): 251–53.

189 Only twenty-two states require the vaccine for school enrollment. In a 2001 survey, 50 percent of parents preferred. Privately funded study released on 6 August 2001 by the National Association of Pediatric Nurse Practitioners (Cherry Hill, N.J.), *Chickenpox Alert: An Estimated Three Million Children Head to School Unvaccinated, Risking Serious Complications.*

190 there was an outbreak of nineteen cases in the Dominican Republic. Centers for Disease Control and Prevention, "Outbreak of poliomyelitis—Dominican Republic and Haiti, 2000–2001," *Journal of the American Medical Association* 285.11 (2001): 1438.

191 Mathematical models show that varicella vaccine coverage must approach 90 percent. M. E. Halloran et al., "Theoretical epidemiologic and morbidity effects of routine varicella immunization of preschool children in the United States," *American Journal of Epidemiology* 140.2 (1994): 81–104.

191 As the American Academy of Pediatrics asserts, "[Physicians] who withhold varicella immunization." American Academy of Pediatrics, "Varicella vaccine update," cited above.

191 In 1888, a German physician noted that children like Patrick developed chickenpox. E. Bruusgaard, "The mutual relation between zoster and varicella," *British Journal of Dermatology and Syphilology* 44 (1932): 1; M. L. McCrary, J. Severson, and S. K. Tyring, "Varicella zoster virus," *Journal of the American Academy of Dermatology* 41.1 (1999): 1–14.

192 In addition, preliminary data suggest that the vaccine also decreases the risk of shingles. A. Gershon and S. Silverstein, "Live attenuated varicella vaccine for prevention of herpes zoster," *Biologicals* 25.2 (1997): 227–30.

7. GONADS

197 only half felt comfortable initiating such a discussion. L. A. Rawitscher, R. Saitz, and L. S. Friedman, "Adolescents'

preferences regarding human immunodeficiency virus (HIV)–related physician counseling and HIV testing," *Pediatrics* 96.1, pt. 1 (1995): 52–58.

197   85 percent of parents wanted their children to get information on safe sex.   R. M. Cavanaugh, Jr. et al., "Anticipatory guidance for the adolescent. Parents' concerns," *Clinical Pediatrics* 32.9 (1993): 542–45.

197   three-quarters report having had intercourse at least once. Centers for Disease Control and Prevention, "Trends in sexual risk behaviors among high school students—United States, 1991–1997," *Morbidity and Mortality Weekly Report* 47.36 (1998): 749–52.

197   one-third of students describing themselves as virgins had engaged in masturbation with an opposite sex partner, and 10 percent had performed oral sex.   M. A. Schuster, R. M. Bell, and D. E. Kanouse, "The sexual practices of adolescent virgins: genital sexual activities of high school students who have never had vaginal intercourse," *American Journal of Public Health* 86.11 (1996): 1570–76.

197   a structured interviewing method called Getting into Adolescents' HEADSS.   E. Cohen, R. G. Mackenzie, and G. L. Yates, "HEADSS, a psychosocial risk assessment instrument: implications for designing effective intervention programs for runaway youth," *Journal of Adolescent Health* 12.7 (1991): 539–44.

198   One in ten female teens having sex carry chlamydia, a common venereal disease, and about a third of teenagers have ridden in a car with an intoxicated driver.   M. A. Gevelber and F. M. Biro, "Adolescents and sexually transmitted diseases," *Pediatric Clinics of North America* 46.4 (1999): 747–66.

199   is at risk of unhealthy alcohol use and needs further assessment. J. R. Knight et al., "Reliabilities of short substance abuse screening tests among adolescent medical patients," *Pediatrics* 105.4, pt. 2 (2000): 948–53.

199   One to 2 percent of high schoolers view themselves as mostly or completely homosexual, and fully 10 percent are unsure.

G. Remafedi et al., "Demography of sexual orientation in adolescents," *Pediatrics* 89.4, pt. 2 (1992): 714–21.

200   Like about half of teens.   F. L. Sonenstein, J. H. Pleck, and L. C. Ku, "Sexual activity, condom use and AIDS awareness among adolescent males," *Family Planning Perspectives* 21.4 (1989): 152–58.

200   Fewer than one in ten males has ever received medical instruction.   Centers for Disease Control and Prevention, "HIV prevention practices of primary-care physicians—United States, 1992," *Journal of the American Medical Association* 271.4 (1994): 261–62.

200   males report that their condom broke during intercourse over the past year.   L. D. Lindberg et al., "Young men's experience with condom breakage," *Family Planning Perspectives* 29.3 (1997): 128–31, 140.

200   teens with available condoms are three times more likely to use them consistently.   R. W. Hingson et al., "Beliefs about AIDS, use of alcohol and drugs, and unprotected sex among Massachusetts adolescents," *American Journal of Public Health* 80.3 (1990): 295–99.

200   scaring teens about AIDS hasn't been shown to improve condom use.   D. P. Orr and C. D. Langefeld, "Factors associated with condom use by sexually active male adolescents at risk for sexually transmitted disease," *Pediatrics* 91.5 (1993): 873–79.

201   an epidemic of breast development among Italian schoolboys. G. M. Fara et al., "Epidemic of breast enlargement in an Italian school," *Lancet* 2.8137 (1979): 295–97.

202   growth may be caused by certain antifungal medications or excessive marijuana smoking.   Jean D. Wilson and Daniel W. Foster, *Williams Textbook of Endocrinology*, 8th ed. (Philadelphia: W. B. Saunders, 1992).

203   40 percent of patients with the problem died; today, only 5 percent succumb to it.   S. Kinkade, "Testicular cancer," *American Family Physician* 59.9 (1999): 2539–44, 2549–50 is a good review of the diagnosis and prognosis associated with testicular cancer.

205   "there is nothing in the between but getting wenches with child." William Shakespeare, *The Winter's Tale*, in New Folger Library

Shakespeare Series, ed. Paul Werstine, act III, scene iii (New York: Washington Square Press, 1998).

205   about *one in ten* American girls between the ages of fifteen and nineteen gets pregnant every year, and 90 percent of these are unintended.   S. J. Ventura et al., "Trends in pregnancies and pregnancy rates by outcome: estimates for the United States, 1976–96," *Vital and Health Statistics* 21.56 (2000): 1–47. Several statistics from this source are used in this section.

205   slightly over a third of these pregnant teens end up getting abortions.   M. Polaneczky and K. O'Connor, "Pregnancy in the adolescent patient. Screening, diagnosis, and initial management," *Pediatric Clinics of North America* 46.4 (1999): 649–70.

206   then "activate" gestation by "penetrating" the egg.   Emily Martin, *The Woman in the Body: A Cultural Analysis of Reproduction* (Boston: Beacon Press, 1987).

206   over twenty-five years and is considered about 75 percent effective.   L. H. Schilling, "Awareness of the existence of postcoital contraception among students who have had a therapeutic abortion," *Journal of American College Health* 32.6 (1984): 244–46.

206   mention its existence to adolescents during routine checkups.   A. Glasier, "Emergency postcoital contraception," *New England Journal of Medicine* 337.15 (1997): 1058–64.

207   a budding gynecologist named Homer Wells, refuses to perform an abortion.   John Irving, *The Cider House Rules* (New York: Ballantine Books, 1996).

208   occurs legally twenty-six million times a year in the world and twenty million times a year illegally.   Abortion statistics derived from "Abortion in fact: Levels, trends, and patterns," *Sharing Responsibility: Women, Society, and Abortion Worldwide* (New York: Alan Guttmacher Institute, 1999): 25–31. Several statistics from this source were used in this section.

209   86 percent of counties have no abortion providers or facilities.   S. K. Henshaw, "Abortion incidence and services in the United States, 1995–1996," *Family Planning Perspectives* 30.6 (1998): 263–70, 287.

209   RU-486, was approved over a decade ago in France and caused no increase on that country's abortion rates. S. Christin-Maitre, P. Bouchard, and I. M. Spitz, "Medical termination of pregnancy," *New England Journal of Medicine* 342.13 (2000): 946–56. This is a comprehensive discussion about oral medications that induce abortions.

209   percentages of American teens that abort are 33, 200, and 500 higher. Malcolm Gladwell, "Operation Rescue," *The New Yorker*, 17 September 2001. Citing this data, Gladwell argues that sex education, not restricting access, could reduce abortion rates.

211   there were one hundred and fifty-six acts of intercourse, but only five references to contraception. B. Greenberg and R. Busselle, "Soap opera and sexual activity: a decade later," *Journal of Communication* 46 (1996): 153–60.

211   contains an average of eight sexual incidents, a fourfold increase from 1976. D. Kunkel, K. Cope, and C. Colvin, *Sexual Messages on Family Hour Television: Content and Context* (Los Angeles: Children Now, 1996).

211   14,000 sexual references per year of which only 1 percent deal with sexually transmitted diseases, pregnancy, or contraception. L. Harris, *Sexual Material on American Network Television during the 1987–1988 Season* (New York: Planned Parenthood Federation of America, 1988); D. Lowry and J. Shidler, "Prime-time TV portrayals of sex, 'safe' sex, and AIDS: a longitudinal analysis," *Journalism Quarterly* 70 (1993): 628–37.

211   one-third of schools have no sex education at all . . . contraceptive information either prohibited or limited to describing lack of efficacy. American Academy of Pediatrics: Committee on Psychosocial Aspects of Child and Family Health and Committee on Adolescence. "Sexuality education for children and adolescents," *Pediatrics* 108.2 (2001): 498–502.

212   Thought to have originated over six thousand years ago . . . and other groups. S. E. Lerman and J. C. Liao, "Neonatal circumcision," *Pediatric Clinics of North America* 48.6 (2001): 1539–57. A

comprehensive review of the history and methods used for circumcision.

212   claiming its therapeutic role in gout, asthma, alcohol dependence, seizures, and other conditions.   P. C. Remondino, *History of Circumcision from the Earliest Times to the Present* (Philadelphia: F. A. Davis, 1891).

212   In 1997, a team of Canadian researchers led by Gideon Koren. A. Taddio et al., "Efficacy and safety of lidocaine-prilocaine cream for pain during circumcision," *New England Journal of Medicine* 336.17 (1997): 1197–201.

213   Circumcision had recently fallen into disfavor.   S. E. Lerman and J. C. Liao, cited above.

214   "parents should determine what is in the best interest of the child." American Academy of Pediatrics Task Force on Circumcision, "Circumcision policy statement," *Pediatrics* 103.3 (1999): 686–93.

214   speaking for a group of avowed foes of the AAP's position.   E. J. Schoen, T. E. Wiswell, and S. Moses, "New policy on circumcision—cause for concern," *Pediatrics* 105.3, pt. 1 (2000): 620–23.

214   Nahid Toubia, a surgeon with extensive experience in Sudan. N. Toubia, "Female circumcision as a public health issue," *New England Journal of Medicine* 331.11 (1994): 712–16.

219   after growing up as a teen girl decided to live as an adult man. John Colapinto, *As Nature Made Him: The Boy Who Was Raised as a Girl* (New York: HarperCollins, 2000).

219   Lacking normal 5-alpha-reductase in their developing genitals. J. Imperato-McGinley et al., "Steroid 5-alpha-reductase deficiency in man: an inherited form of male pseudohermaphroditism," *Science* 186.4170 (1974): 1213–15.

220   Biochemist Joseph Goldstein calls it.   Michael Brown and Joseph Goldstein, from their 1985 Nobel Prize acceptance speech, "A receptor-mediated pathway for cholesterol homeostasis." The full text is available at http://www.nobel.se/medicine/laureates/1985/goldstein-lecture.html.

221   In 1975, Anke Ehrhardt compared seventeen patients.   Anke

Ehrhardt, "Prenatal hormone exposure and psychosexual differentiation," in *Topics in Psychoendocrinology*, ed. E. J. Sachar (New York: Grune & Stratton, 1975).

222   40 percent of adult women with CAH said they were "exclusively heterosexual," and that 35 percent were "bisexual or homosexual."   J. Money, M. Schwartz, and V. G. Lewis, "Adult erotosexual status and fetal hormonal masculinization and demasculinization: 46,XX congenital virilizing adrenal hyperplasia and 46,XY androgen-insensitivity syndrome compared," *Psychoneuroendocrinology* 9.4 (1984): 405–14. In his later papers, such as this one, John Money advocated a role for prenatal hormone exposure in determining sexual identity.

8. GUTS

225   The mystery of how flour mixed with water becomes dough. K. A. Tilley et al., "Tyrosine cross-links: molecular basis of gluten structure and function," *Journal of Agricultural and Food Chemistry* 49.5 (2001): 2627–32.

227   Generally, the average infant passes a half-teaspoon's worth. L. T. Weaver, "Bowel habit from birth to old age," *Journal of Pediatric Gastroenterology and Nutrition* 7.5 (1988): 637–40; J. A. Goy et al., "Fecal characteristics contrasted in the irritable bowel syndrome and diverticular disease," *American Journal of Clinical Nutrition* 29.12 (1976): 1480–84.

227   about two and a half gallons of fluid enter the average child's duodenum.   J. S. Fordtran and T. W. Locklear, "Ionic constituents and osmolality of gastric and small-intestinal fluids after eating," *American Journal of Digestive Disease* 11.7 (1966): 503–21.

227   the food travels through the twelve feet of the small intestine. J. M. Nightingale, C. I. Bartram, and J. E. Lennard-Jones, "Length of residual small bowel after partial resection: correlation between radiographic and surgical measurements," *Gastrointestinal Radiology* 16.4 (1991): 305–6.

227   and 90 percent of the water are absorbed.   S. F. Phillips and
      J. Giller, "The contribution of the colon to electrolyte and water
      conservation in man," *Journal of Laboratory and Clinical Medicine*
      81.5 (1973): 733–46.

228   villi that expand the surface area of the small intestine.
      S. Tabrez and I. M. Roberts, "Malabsorption and malnutrition,"
      Primary Care 28.3 (2001): 505–22.

228   The great physician William Osler called.   W. Osler, *The
      Principles and Practice of Medicine* (New York: D. Appleton, 1892).

228   a *single gram* of feces from an infected person.   D. Acheson and
      G. Keusch, "Shigella and enteroinvasive Escherichia coli," in
      Infections of the Gastrointestinal Tract, ed. M. Blaser et al. (New York:
      Raven Press, 1995) 763–84.

229   the well-appearing Irish immigrant Mary Mallon.   G. Soper,
      "Curious career of Typhoid Mary," *Bulletin of the New York
      Academy of Medicine* 15 (1939).

229   in Wasco County, Oregon, it was used in history's first bioterror-
      ist attack.   T. J. Torok et al., "A large community outbreak of
      salmonellosis caused by intentional contamination of restau-
      rant salad bars," *Journal of the American Medical Association* 278.5
      (1997): 389–95.

229   source from which Iraqi agents may have obtained anthrax.
      Laurie Garrett, *Betrayal of Trust: The Collapse of Global Public Health*
      (New York: Hyperion, 2000).

229   the U.S. Department of Agriculture reports that 30 percent of
      ground turkey and 15 percent of ground chicken.   U.S. Depart-
      ment of Agriculture Food Safety and Inspection Service, "HACCP
      Implementation: Salmonella Compliance Test Results, January
      26, 1998 to January 24, 2000." Available at http://www.fsis.usda.
      gov/ophs/haccp/salcomp.pdf, accessed March 8, 2002.

229   children developed *Salmonella* infection after petting a Komodo
      dragon.   C. R. Friedman et al., "An outbreak of salmonellosis
      among children attending a reptile exhibit at a zoo," *Journal of
      Pediatrics* 132.5 (1998): 802–7.

229   undercooked hamburgers made by the Jack-in-the-Box.   B. P. Bell et al., "A multistate outbreak of Escherichia coli O157:H7-associated bloody diarrhea and hemolytic uremic syndrome from hamburgers: the Washington experience," *Journal of the American Medical Association* 272.17 (1994): 1349–53.

230   About 2 percent of children have allergies to cow's milk.   J. M. Spergel and N. A. Pawlowski, "Food allergy: mechanisms, diagnosis, and management in children," *Pediatric Clinics of North America* 49.1 (2002): 73–96.

230   In these individuals, lactose passes whole.   J. R. Saltzman and R. M. Russell, "The aging gut: nutritional issues," *Gastroenterology Clinics of North America* 27.2 (1998): 309–24.

230   reports of operating-room explosions during gastrointestinal surgery in lactose intolerant people.   F. S. Joyce and T. N. Rasmussen, "Gas explosion during diathermy gastrotomy," *Gastroenterology* 96.2, pt. 1 (1989): 530–31.

231   the most common cause of diarrhea in children today.   K. Ramaswamy and K. Jacobson, "Infectious diarrhea in children," *Gastroenterology Clinics of North America* 30.3 (2001): 611–24.

231   about $300 in extra day-care costs and lost wages.   P. Avendano et al., "Costs associated with office visits for diarrhea in infants and toddlers," *Pediatric Infectious Disease Journal* 12.11 (1993): 897–902.

231   Every year, 200,000 American infants are hospitalized for diarrhea and 500 die.   R. I. Glass et al., "Estimates of morbidity and mortality rates for diarrheal diseases in American children," *Journal of Pediatrics* 118.4, pt. 2 (1991): S27–33.

231   Cholera originated in areas around India's Ganges River.   G. Keusch and R. Deresiewicz, "Cholera and other vibrioses," in *Harrison's Principles of Internal Medicine*, ed. K. Isselbacher et al., 13th ed. (New York: McGraw-Hill, 1994).

231   seven global pandemics of cholera have occurred.   Ibid.

232   In Malaysia, an interesting discovery was made.   P. S. Rao et al., "Intravenous administration of coconut water," *Journal of the Association of Physicians of India* 203 (1972): 235–39.

232   In the 1950s, doctors figured that a beverage with the same salt.
H. E. Harrison, "The treatment of diarrhea in infancy," *Pediatric
Clinics of North America* 1 (1954): 335–48.

232   In 1964, R. Phillips found that glucose.   R. A. Phillips, "Water
and electrolyte losses in cholera," *Federation Proceedings* 23 (1964):
705–12.

232   In the mid-1970s, the World Health Organization agreed.
This decision was made largely due to a landmark study, N.
Hirschhorn et al., "Decrease in net stool output in cholera dur-
ing intestinal perfusion with glucose-containing solutions,"
New England Journal of Medicine 279.4 (1968): 176–81.

232   A homemade recipe for ORS.   G. Keusch and R. Deresiewicz,
"Cholera and other vibrioses," cited above.

233   fatality rates from cholera epidemics fell dramatically.   P. Shears,
"Cholera," *Annals of Tropical Medicine and Parasitology* 88.2 (1994):
109–22.

233   At his first meeting with tribal officials, he was asked.
Mathuram Santosham, *Contributions of American Indian Populations
in Controlling Infectious Disease*, Grand Rounds lecture at Children's
Hospital, Boston, 15 October 1997.

233   In a 1985 study in Whiteriver, Arizona, Santosham.   M. Santosham et al., "Oral rehydration therapy for acute diarrhea in
ambulatory children in the United States: a double-blind comparison of four different solutions," *Pediatrics* 76.2 (1985): 159–66.

233   chicken broth has twice as much salt.   Electrolyte concentra-
tion of clear liquids are from R. H. Squires, "Management of
Diarrhea," in *Pediatric Gastrointestinal Disease*, ed. R. Wyllie and
J. S. Hyams, 2d ed. (Philadelphia: W. B. Saunders, 1999).

234   regular diet should be resumed.   American Academy of Pediatrics, "Practice parameter: the management of acute gastro-
enteritis in young children," *Pediatrics* 97.3 (1996): 424–35.

236   Thousands of years ago, ancient Hindu physicians described a
strange, deadly condition.   Information regarding the history
of diabetes and the discovery of insulin are from J. MacCracken
and D. Hoel, "From ants to analogues: puzzles and promises in

diabetes management," *Postgraduate Medicine* 101.4 (1997): 138–40, 143–45, 149–50.

237   the condition affecting folk musician Woody Guthrie.   Eric Goldscheider, "At Home with Arlo Guthrie," *Boston Globe*, 22 November 2001.

237   "devil you know is far better than the one you don't."   Richard Saltus, "Genetic clairvoyance," *Boston Globe Sunday Magazine*, 8 January 1995.

237   Ergun Uc, an Arkansas specialist.   John Haman, "The small Arkansas world of a terrible genetic disease," *Arkansas Times*, 16 April 1999.

238   a rat poison called Vacor was pulled from the market.   P. A. LeWitt, "The neurotoxicity of the rat poison vacor: a clinical study of 12 cases," *New England Journal of Medicine* 302.2 (1980): 73–77.

242   In 1969, psychiatrist Elisabeth Kübler-Ross.   Elisabeth Kübler-Ross, *On Death and Dying* (New York: Macmillan, 1969).

244   In 1990, for example, a researcher placed a group of obese patients.   R. Lappalainen et al., "Hunger/craving responses and reactivity to food stimuli during fasting and dieting," *International Journal of Obesity* 14.8 (1990): 679–88.

244   In another study on patients with Meg's specific problem.   D. J. Broberg and I. L. Bernstein, "Cephalic insulin release in anorexic women," *Physiology and Behavior* 45.5 (1989): 871–74.

245   surveys show that more than half of all adolescent girls are trying to lose weight.   L. Kann et al., "Youth risk behavior surveillance—United States, 1997," *Morbidity and Mortality Weekly Report* 47.3 (1998): 1–89.

245   80 percent of girls thinking they were too fat actually had normal body weights.   D. B. Woodside, "A review of anorexia nervosa and bulimia nervosa," *Current Problems in Pediatrics* 25.2 (1995): 67–89.

245   if Mattel's Barbie doll were a standard female height.   Ann Ducille, "Dyes and dolls: multicultural Barbie and the merchandising of difference," *Differences: A Journal of Feminist Cultural Studies* 6.1 (1994): 46–67.

245 almost one in ten adolescent girls takes diet pills, and one in five college-age women.   L. Kann et al., "Youth risk behavior surveillance—United States, 1997," cited above.

246 In his memoir *A Leg to Stand On*, neurologist Oliver Sacks.   Oliver W. Sacks, *A Leg to Stand On* (New York: Summit Books, 1984).

247 In the 1940s, concentration camp survivors and prisoners of war.   S. M. Solomon and D. F. Kirby, "The refeeding syndrome: a review," *Journal of Parenteral and Enteral Nutrition* 14.1 (1990): 90–97.

247 American volunteers in the 1940s fasted for several weeks and then began eating.   A. Keys, "Cardiovascular effects of malnutrition and starvation," *Modern Concepts of Cardiovascular Disease* 27 (1948): 21.

249 A proposed—though controversial—risk factor.   A. D. Schwabe et al., "Anorexia nervosa," *Annals of Internal Medicine* 94 (1981): 371–81.

249 "shouting and unrelenting 'No,' which extends to every area of living."   H. Bruch, "Developmental considerations of anorexia nervosa and obesity," *Canadian Journal of Psychiatry* 26 (1981): 212–17.

249 anorexic patients "seem to be retreating further into childhood."   R. E. Kreipe and S. A. Birndorf, "Eating disorders in adolescents and young adults," *Medical Clinics of North America* 84.4 (2000): 1027–49.

250 binges of up to 50,000 calories in a day.   J. E. Mitchell, R. L. Pyle, and E. D. Eckert, "Frequency and duration of binge-eating episodes in patients with bulimia," *American Journal of Psychiatry* 138 (1981): 835–36.

250 "I go on eating after I've satisfied [normal] hunger."   G. Russell, "Bulimia nervosa: an ominous variant of anorexia nervosa," *Psychological Medicine* 9 (1979): 429–48.

250 one in ten, eventually die of starvation.   D. B. Herzog, K. M. Nussbaum, and A. K. Marmor, "Comorbidity and outcome in eating disorders," *Psychiatry Clinics of North America* 19.4 (1996): 843–59.

ACKNOWLEDGMENTS

This book—like many others—resulted from a coincidence. During my internship at Children's Hospital, Boston, I began writing an essay on the case of Matthew Eappen. One of the individuals I interviewed, Eli Newberger, was taking a sabbatical year off to write a book on the psychology of adolescent boys. He introduced me to his agent, Donald Cutler, who took me on as a bit of a charity case. He quickly became my cheerleader and most valued critic. Donald's coaxing finally convinced me that I really could write a book about children. I still had a lot to learn: When we met a publisher for lunch, I gauchely ordered a messy plate of ribs and ate like the famished medical resident I was. All the more gratitude then goes to Jack Macrae at Henry Holt, who signed me anyway. After my father died unexpectedly, Jack patiently gave me all the extra time I needed to complete the project. His gentle touch was ideal for both the book and me. I also thank his assistant Katy Hope, who carefully handled many details regarding the manuscript.

Almost seventeen years ago, I luckily took a class given by Matthew Carr, who ignited a continuing passion for writing. At a series of seminars, Verlyn Klinkenborg (now at the *New York Times*) helped refine that passion a few years later.

I am grateful to Gail Boaz, Jeff Camp, Joan and Arnold Chait, Maria Farnon, Annie Kessler, Kerry Parsons, Merle Price, and Joe Ronayne for their insightful comments on early portions of the book. My sister, Mita Goel, retrieved numerous articles for me from the Countway Library at Harvard Medical School. Dick Krugman sent me several technical publications and gave his time generously, despite the demands of being the dean of the University of Colorado medical center. My old friend Beth Croce drew a series of wonderful illustrations at short notice.

In memory of their son Matthew, Sunil and Deborah Eappen established an annual Children's Hospital educational grant, which I used to attend an enlightening workshop on the diagnosis and management of child abuse. To them and all the children and families about whom I wrote, I owe more than I can say. Thank you for allowing me into your lives.

After my father died, my mother, Rita Sanghavi, by her example, taught me the importance of embracing life even in the wake of sorrow. Finally, I am indebted to my wife, Elizabeth, who read draft after draft of the book, took care of our infant son night after late night while I wrote, and has always been unwavering in her confidence in me. My love for her is limitless.

INDEX

294   INDEX

ABOUT THE AUTHOR

DARSHAK SANGHAVI attended medical school at Johns Hopkins University and served his residency at Harvard's Children's Hospital in Boston. He has done medical research in rural Appalachia, Japan, Kenya, and Peru, and recently worked for the U.S. Indian Health Service on a Navajo reservation in New Mexico. Now training in pediatric cardiology at Children's Hospital, he lives near Boston with his wife and son.